FINDING STRENGTH TO LIVE
WITH ILLNESS

Bridge To Healing

ISRAELA MEYERSTEIN

Mazo Publishers

Bridge To Healing

ISBN: 978-1-936778-48-5 – Soft Cover (Paper)
ISBN: 978-1-936778-20-1 – Hard Cover (Cloth)

Email: israela.meyerstein@gmail.com
Website: www.bridge-to-healing.com

Library of Congress Control Number: 2014947903
Subject matter:
Healing; Spirituality; Cancer; Judaism; Mind and Body;
Holistic and Integrative Medicine

Published by
Mazo Publishers
P.O. Box 10474 ~ Jacksonville, FL 32247 USA
USA: 1-815-301-3559

Website: www.mazopublishers.com
Email: mazopublishers@gmail.com

Cover Design: Studio ERachel
Front Cover Image: © Nadia Starovoitova ⊦ Dreamstime

The author and publisher have made every effort to provide accurate information in this book. However, they are not responsible for the outcomes related to the use of the contents of this book, or the procedures described, which may not be applicable to all people. Specific treatment for health matters should administered under the direction of your health care provider.

Contents

Endorsements

"Bridge To Healing" is just what the title implies. Healing and curing are two distinct entities. I have learned that when you heal your life, your body gets a live message and does all it can to help you to survive.

Cancer is a unique experience for each individual. When you are willing to explore your experience and ask what you are to learn from your journey through Hell, the curse can become a blessing; just as hunger makes us seek nourishment, so can our disease.

Israela shares some of the universal themes one can find in many religions and philosophies which have proven to be effective. She shows us how to heal, find peace, and not wage a war against the cancer enemy and empower it. She shows us how to treat the experience and not just the result.

Israela removes the guilt, shame and blame issues, and like Maimonides, understands that disease is not God's punishment. What you need to do is seek help by looking for what you have lost: your health. I have seen self-induced healing occur when people had faith, left their troubles to God, and had their cancers disappear. I have learned from exceptional patients about survivor behavior.

God loves His children and our healing potential is amazing. So read on and learn from the wisdom of the sages and ages that you are not a diagnosis or a statistic. You are a survivor.

Bernie S. Siegel, M.D.
Author of 365 Prescriptions for the Soul:
Daily Messages of Inspiration, Hope, and Love

We all face the prospect of serious illness in our lives and how we learn and cope with this crisis is an essential human task. "Bridge To Healing" by Israela Meyerstein is more than an inspiring tale of illness and recovery; it guides us through the process of loss of health and its recovery utilizing spiritual tools that are specific and useful. Inspired by Jewish tradition, it has universal appeal as its wisdom comes from the ages.

Steven S. Sharfstein, M.D.
President and CEO
Sheppard Pratt Health System, Maryland

I commend your dedication to cover the topic so thoroughly.
Rabbi Harold S. Kushner

"Bridge To Healing" is one of the most inspiring journeys through personal illness I have read in years. I cannot imagine anyone who will not benefit from the practical methods that psychotherapist Israela Meyerstein devised to survive and thrive following her encounter with cancer. This is a marvelous account of the power of spirituality in enduring life's greatest challenges. It is also a work of great compassion, for it will lighten the burden of illness not only for the sufferer, but also for those who care for them.
Larry Dossey, M.D.
Author of *One Mind: How Our Individual Mind Is Part of a Greater Consciousness and Why It Matters*

Drawing on her profound experiences as a gifted family therapist, searching cancer patient, and thoughtful student/facilitator of spiritual growth, Israela Meyerstein has constructed a sturdy and beautiful bridge to healing for patients, caregiving family and friends, health care professionals, and, truly, all those touched by our precarious human condition. Her personal and professional voices are artfully integrated and join a chorus of Jewish and many other texts of coping and hoping, providing both deeply inspiring and remarkably practical guidance and tools for the journeys of illness, recovery, and healing.
Rabbi Simkha Y. Weintraub, LCSW,
Rabbinic Director, National Center for Jewish Healing
and New York Jewish Healing Center;
Jewish Board of Family and Children's Services

Israela Meyerstein's book on Practical Spirituality builds from her own experiences as a cancer survivor. Her story of battling disease is extraordinary in her development and sharing of tools – she finds a path to stay actively human, not simply a passive patient in a dehumanized technical battle for her body. Many other people will find themselves, or someone they love, in a similar struggle. Israela's sharing of her experiences, and tools she found useful, can help bring light and hope to a stressful journey.
Harold Bob, M.D., C.M.D.
Medical Director, Seasons Hospice, Maryland

The theme of the subtitle of this book, Finding Strength To Cope With Illness, is an inspiration for patients, caregivers, and health care professionals. What makes it authentic is Israela Meyerstein's personal journey through the disempowering complex labyrinth of oncology. What makes it truly practical for anyone are the spiritual resources that have their roots in Judaism, but are universal in nature. The message is clear: We can overcome the many challenging aspects of cancer when we step outside the limits of disease-centered medicine (where the heart is seen as a pump) and enter the realm of individualized, human-centered medicine (where the heart connects with the spirit). Israela's book, "Bridge To Healing", is the roadmap to get there.

Peter Hinderberger, M.D., Ph.D., DI Hom. Medical Director
Ruscombe Mansion Community Health Center Baltimore, Maryland

Sensitivity, Spirituality, and Israela are one and the same. As a gifted psychotherapist she has helped numerous people find peace and direction within themselves. As Israela points out, many who are confronted with illness and other life challenges either begin to use or lose religion. Challenges that "cut a hole in the soul" can also reawaken a search for purpose in life. Writing from personal experience with illness, Israela shows readers how spirituality can bring renewed strength and positive hope for the future. Follow her journey and you, too, will find renewed strength to cope and heal!

Rabbi Dr. Tsvi G. Schur
Chaplain, Johns Hopkins Hospital

"Bridge To Healing" is more than "just" a health care book with Jewish and universal appeal; it is an inspirational guide to improve your life. Israela demonstrates that she is just as conversant with Judaic sources as she is with spiritual and wellness literature. I was moved by the breadth and depth of her thinking and lively style. Self-help guides don't get any better than this!

Rabbi Dr. Ed Weinsberg
Author of *Conquer Prostate Cancer:
How Medicine, Faith, Love, and Sex Can Renew Your Life*

Israela's story is both riveting and uplifting. Israela enables readers to trust her as their guide.

Rabbi Nina Beth Cardin
Author of *Tears of Sorrow, Seeds of Hope*

Acknowledgments

My illness journey made gratitude my strongest emotion. The Hebrew words, "*hakarat hatov*" mean "recognition of the good." I have many people to whom I owe thanks, starting with the wonderful doctors, nurses, and professionals who guided me back to health. Their skill and caring made them true partners with God in my healing.

Having a supportive family made all the difference in my being able to focus my energy and strength on coping with the important challenge I faced. I was not alone, but rather surrounded by a caring circle of my *chavurah* – friendship group – and special friends who came forward to provide practical help and emotional support in my time of need.

I am indebted to The National Center for Jewish Healing under the creative spiritual leadership of Rabbi Simkha Y. Weintraub for the inspiration to co-lead groups for patients facing serious medical illness.

My rich collaboration with friend and colleague, Rabbi Gila Ruskin, led to our developing spiritual resources for patients which later helped me cope with my own ordeal.

Some say "it takes a village" to cope with illness. I found that it also takes a village to publish a book, and many people were instrumental in its development from conception to birth.

I am grateful to Dr. Peter Hinderberger and Rabbi Tzvi Hersh Weinreb for believing in the merit of the book early on.

I also thank Rabbi Ron Shulman, Rabbi Nina B. Cardin, Dr. Bernie Siegel, Rabbi Harold S. Kushner, Dr. Larry Dossey, Dr. Salvador Minuchin, Garry Cooper, Dr. Gail and M. Hirsh Goldberg, Claudia Simpson, Lynn Stewart, Judy Haiduk, Wendy Minnix, Judy Meltzer, and Joan Katz for their participation.

For tremendous encouragement and giving generously of their time to carefully read and sometimes re-read entire versions of the manuscript and offer constructive feedback, I am most grateful to Danny Siegel, Dr. Steve S. Sharfstein, Dr. Harold Bob, Rabbi Dr. Tsvi G. Schur, Dr. Paul and Rabbi Gila Ruskin, Chaplain Maureen O'Brien, Rabbi Jim Michaels, Betty Pristera,

Golda Jacobs, Louise Alima, and Margie Koretzky.

I am very grateful to Chaim Mazo at Mazo Publishers who provided expert advice and editorial support in an efficient, flexible, and most personable, professional manner.

Additional editorial help and encouragement came from Martha Murphy, Barbara Trainin Blank, and Rabbi Ed Weinsberg.

My husband Michael stood lovingly by my side, giving excellent editorial support and encouraging my efforts and persistence. As with illness, it would have been too hard to go it alone.

About The Author

Israela Meyerstein, LCSW-C, LCMFT, has been helping families, couples, and individuals for forty years, treating a variety of problems, including parenting and family relationships, couple issues, coping with separation, divorce, and remarriage, medical illness, fetal loss, spirituality and healthy personal coping. In private practice since 1978, she was recognized in 2001 as a leading mental health professional by Baltimore Magazine.

Israela Meyerstein completed her MSW degree in 1973 from Columbia University School of Social Work, followed by a Third Year Fellowship in Social Work at the University of Texas Medical Branch in Galveston, Texas, where she was later appointed Faculty Associate in the Division of Community and Social Psychiatry of the Medical School.

An Approved Supervisor in the American Association for Marriage and Family Therapy, Ms. Meyerstein directed a Family Therapy Training Program at Sheppard Pratt Hospital from 1986-1998. She has trained hundreds of professionals of varied disciplines, and has taught Family Therapy in college and graduate level programs.

Israela co-founded the Baltimore Jewish Healing Network. Together with Rabbi Gila Ruskin, she co-led Spiritual Study/ Discussion groups for those struggling with medical illness. Ms. Meyerstein has authored thirty published articles on couples and family therapy, spirituality, medical illness, remarriage, and therapist training. "Bridge To Healing: Finding Strength To Cope With Illness" is her first book.

"A small hole in the body produces a greater hole in the soul."

Yiddish saying

"Know! A person walks in life on a very narrow bridge. The most important thing is not to be afraid."

Reb Nachman of Breslov
Likutey Moharan 11:48

Stems Out Of Scratches

*A king once owned a large, beautiful, flawless gem,
of which he was justifiably very proud,
for it had no equivalent anywhere in the world.*

*One day, the gem dropped and acquired a deep scratch.
The king summoned the most highly skilled jewelers and offered a
great reward for anyone who could remove the imperfection from
his treasured jewel.*

*But alas, none could repair the damaged gem, and the king was
deeply depressed.*

*After some time, a gifted lapidary came to the king and promised
to make the rare gem even more beautiful than before the mishap.
The king, impressed with this expert's confidence, entrusted his
precious stone to his care.*

*With superb artistry, the craftsman engraved a lovely rosebud
around the imperfection – the scratch now becoming a strong and
graceful stem of the flower.*

*Some say the king balked at first,
but soon renewed his
appreciation for his treasure,
which now embodied, not only its past beauty,*
but new possibilities and directions.[1]

Introduction

In the opening scene of the play *Man of La Mancha,* a prisoner of the Spanish Inquisition named Miguel de Cervantes is thrown into a dungeon, where he faces the terror of an uncertain fate. To cope with his imprisonment Cervantes creates an imaginative drama about Don Quixote, the idealistic knight who chases windmills using his heart for navigation, and endures scorn for seeing beauty where others cannot. Cervantes enlists his fellow inmates to play the various roles and brings the adventure to life with music, humor, and fantasy. For a brief time the drama distracts the prisoners from their painful fate.

As one of the entranced theatergoers witnessing this play within a play, I realized that Cervantes' creative expression not only helped him transcend his circumstances by lifting mood, offering hope, and creating meaning, but it also moved his fellow prisoners and the theater audience with a message of human resilience, love, and salvation. This favorite drama of mine spoke to me in new ways during an ordeal with illness. It was my personal imprisonment.

This is how it happened to me. In an instant the gynecologist's phone call etched an indelible message on my mind: "The biopsy looks bad. Some mixed type. Everything needs to come out. We should get you into surgery as soon as possible." These few words suddenly transported me on an express train from the land of the well to the land of the sick. Malignancy invaded my body and I became a prisoner, unable to flee.

A sudden and scary diagnosis is only the first stage of an illness experience that throws a person off balance and creates a major detour in life. Each subsequent stage requires new adaptations and a recalibration of who we are and what we still can do in life. Overwhelmed by confusion and fear, I numbly followed the detour sign off my life path into the unfamiliar labyrinth of medical treatment.

I felt as if I had stumbled into a vast wilderness without a map, iPhone, or working GPS. Illness felt like being in a long confining tunnel, not knowing if I would emerge or what to expect at the other end. As I focused anxiously on bodily symptoms, my vision narrowed ("tunnel vision") and it was hard to access a wider perspective or options. Sojourning in the land of the sick created isolation and raised perplexing spiritual questions without answers. Moreover, almost all of my energy was needed to just get by.

Chemotherapy and radiation treatment schedules took over my daily life with side effects that created challenges on physical, emotional, and spiritual levels. After treatments, I was wiped out yet couldn't sleep, and I was pretty much down and out the first week after each chemo session. I worried about suppressed immunity and felt uneasy being out socially. I dreaded the long marathon ahead of me and wondered if I would have enough stamina and courage. I had to scramble to find inner and outer resources to avoid sinking into a depressed, victim-like state. I realized that what had just happened to me was that I was kidnapped by a terrorist named "Illness."

As I was swept into the vortex of life as a "patient," my normal world – as a wife, professional therapist, mother – rapidly fell away. No matter how hard I tried to hold onto it, the life I had carefully crafted and deeply loved was dissolving. While I was to discover eventually that surgical and medical treatment would conquer my illness, the hole it had cut in my soul would not be touched by any of these things. I would have to do that healing work myself.

I joined the ranks of millions of ordinary people who face serious medical struggles, as illness and injury play no favorites in attacking all age, socioeconomic, ethnic, and religious groups. According to a study, one in two men and one in three women in the United States will be diagnosed with cancer in their lifetimes,[1] and over 130 million Americans suffer from chronic conditions.[2] Millions struggle with injury and loss, including the over 45,000 troops plagued with continuing physical wounds and emotional trauma.[3] Over 65 million Americans provide care to elderly, disabled, and chronically ill family members,[4] as well as the many health and mental health professionals who compassionately care for these individuals.

Cancer is a frightening disease requiring extensive and expensive treatments that wear patients out. When our bodies ache, our spirits ache as well. I experienced a range of vulnerable emotions such as anxiety, confusion, helplessness, anger, depression, loneliness, despair, and even guilt, that often accompany illness. Research, however, has found that these emotional states themselves are detrimental to health.[5]

The ripple effects of illness make it a family affair, yet it isn't easy to talk with family members and friends about difficult emotional and spiritual concerns. Spiritual questions such as "Why me?", "Why now?", "What did I do to cause this?", "Is God punishing me?" percolate for many patients as they try to make sense of their plight. Worse yet, many people become disconnected from their spiritual or religious tradition just at a time when they most need comfort and inspiration.

I soon realized that sustaining one's spirits and preserving identity in the face of illness is a daily challenge. It may seem strange to describe the illness or injury as just the tip of the iceberg, but navigating today's complex high tech medical system with its unfamiliar procedures and treatments was an additional stressful job for me. Few people are trained beforehand and there is way too much on-the-job training for patients.

During illness, life often felt on edge, as if standing on a bridge overlooking troubled waters. Reb Nachman reminds us that although we all walk on that narrow bridge of life, we must not succumb to fears that can overwhelm, paralyze, and despair us on our journey. We desperately need a map, a guide, and a repertoire of coping tools and connection to others to help us navigate through this difficult territory and weather the storm of illness. We crave a medicine that will close the hole in the soul that physical malady inevitably creates.

Illness forced me to halt my normal activities but gave me an unexpected gift: time to explore spiritual writings and traditions that are the uniquely human expression of our need to be whole, to connect with Spirit. My spirituality was a rich resource whose words and actions became the medicine that ultimately completed my healing. They were the tools that helped me return to the land of the well.

Holocaust survivor and psychologist Viktor Frankl stated: "Between stimulus and response, there is a space. In that space is our power to choose our response. In our response lies our growth and freedom." I came to believe that how I responded could impact the quality of my life and maybe even the course of illness.

Intuitively at first and then deliberately, I found and gathered these tools, more enlightened and empowered by each one. As I amassed them I began to realize I was creating a toolbox of sorts, a practical means to mend that intangible part of being alive. I turned to wisdom from complementary and alternative approaches (acupuncture, homeopathy, yoga), inspiration from creative expression (art, humor, journaling, music), and comfort from inspirational words, meditation, and nature.

Out of the depths I called to my Jewish tradition. There I found an integrated spiritual perspective and a virtual treasure chest of resources developed over the centuries that address body, mind, and spirit, from the ancient guidelines for visiting the sick to a rich collection of Psalms, prayers, rituals, stories, biblical texts, and *tikkun olam*.

Using any or all of these varied resources can provide psychological benefit to a person struggling with illness or injury. These down-to-earth self-help tools provide an essential component to the healing process. Moreover, these resources can be useful not only during illness, but offer a manifesto for healthy living. Having personally applied these resources I can vouch for their merit, wisdom, and efficacy!

Reconnecting with my inner spirit became the pathway to my healing and renewal. I experienced what the king in the Hasidic parable, *Stems Out Of Scratches*, learned from his ordeal: Out of brokenness, beauty and wholeness that embodies both the past trauma as well as new unfolding possibilities can emerge; surviving serious illness can lead to post-traumatic growth and triumphant thriving.

My illness journey reinforced for me the essential truth of the link between our bodies and our spirit. I remember lying on the gurney just before going into surgery, flanked by my Jewish gynecologist, Moslem gynecological surgeon, and Christian anesthesiologist. I had brought along a prayer to bless the doctors' work and pray for a positive outcome. Although my voice trembled as I read the words, my doctors listened attentively, smiled, and nodded "amen." Perhaps doctors need prayers too. That gesture helped me get ready for the operation. My mind was soothed, my body calmed, and my spirit confident that I was in the hands of a good collaborative team.

My forty years of experience as a clinical social worker helping people, teaching therapists, and writing for professional journals have given me insight about the doctor-patient relationship and what patients need. My personal illness experience offers important lessons to patients, family members and the professionals who care for them. I believe that having a practical spiritual perspective, a map for the journey, and down-to-earth spiritual tools can enable people to navigate their journey more resiliently.

An inspiring story, perhaps an urban myth, is told about the famous violinist, Itzhak Perlman, who was polio-stricken from childhood. He laboriously made his way on stage with crutches to begin a performance. As he started to play, one of his violin strings suddenly popped. The audience froze, wondering what Perlman would do next. Would he leave the stage for a replacement string? The audience waited with bated breath as Perlman picked up his violin and completed the piece with only three strings by constantly readjusting for each note. At the end he received a standing ovation. When asked why he chose to continue despite the loss of the string, he explained that we all have challenges that can devastate us; our task is to continue to play the hand we've been dealt, with what we have left.

Dear Reader, although we have never met, you are a part of my invisible support team. Let me explain. Like a play within a play, I began writing this book as a diary during my "narrow straits" of illness to help me cope with fears, uncertainties, and difficult treatments. Journaling helped me document my experience, acknowledge my emotions, and feel less alone. At times treatment side effects were so debilitating that I couldn't even write, but in the years following treatment my writing gained new meaning and purpose. I welcome the opportunity to share with you the many helpful spiritual coping tools that I used on my illness journey.

Readers of different faiths and beliefs will find valuable healing lessons in this book. All of the varied tools can provide comfort, inspiration, and strengthening. I encourage you to integrate into your life what feels right for you. Creating a practical spiritual toolbox of your very own can make a difference in your coping!

Here is what you can expect as you begin reading:

- Part I introduces you to what I call Practical Spirituality, insights from a Jewish perspective, and my M.A.P.S. approach.
- Part II invites you to follow the diary chronicling my experience as a patient in the medical system. I describe the specific tools I used that helped me in profound ways. I summarize the healing lessons learned and offer practical tips for patients and practitioners.
- Part III describes in more detail the down-to-earth toolbox with its many resources from varied approaches and traditions.
- Part IV gives you an opportunity to examine your own spiritual connections, do a personal spiritual self-assessment, and create a personal spiritual treatment plan.
- Part V provides chapter notes, a glossary, an alphabetical list of reading references and supportive resources.

My illness journey was unlike all others because it was mine. Each illness happens to a different and unique individual. All of us affected by illness, including our caregivers, face challenges on the narrow bridge of life suspended over troubled waters. We are a community of sufferers, survivors, sometimes thrivers … and always human. I hope the healing lessons in this book will comfort and sustain your spirits, lend inspiration, and empower you to strengthen your coping during illness. If they do, then I will have found additional meaning and purpose in writing this book.

PART I
PRACTICAL SPIRITUALITY

Chapter One

What's "Practical Spirituality" Got To Do With Healing?

A Yiddish proverb says it simply: "A small hole in the body produces a greater hole in the soul." In the twentieth century, theologian and social activist Rabbi Abraham Joshua Heschel wrote:

> *"Sickness ... is a crisis of the total person, not only a physical disorder. There is a spiritual dimension to sickness."* [1]

Illness violates our sense of safety and reminds us that life is impermanent, unpredictable, and often unfair.

My body, my companion for almost sixty years, had suddenly betrayed me, stirring up a sandstorm of vulnerable emotions common to the illness experience such as confusion, helplessness, fear, and sadness.

In the trenches of treatment I felt small and alone in the universe, and my craving for support, connection, and inspiration was greater.

No doubt you have heard the saying: "There are no atheists in foxholes," reflecting the human tendency to seek a "Higher Power" when in great danger. This humbling awareness of something bigger invited me to turn to spiritual pathways for healing. Indeed, spirituality and religion may speak louder to us when we are facing disability, incapacitation, or loss in life.

What is Practical Spirituality?

"From where does my help come?" asked the Psalmist long before I wondered how I would pick myself up after being knocked down by illness. How would I find new ways of coping and healing? Practical Spirituality answered my plea by providing me with a spiritual perspective, a map for the territory, and a down-to-earth toolbox for coping.

Perhaps "Practical Spirituality" sounds a little like an oxymoron since "practical" connotes logical, down-to-earth, and functional, while "spirituality" is a matter of the heart, seeking larger meaning and inspiration in life. However, these two disparate aspects can be integrated because Practical Spirituality includes inner reflective experiences of awe as well as behavioral practices, rituals, and community. The "being" (inner reflecting) and "doing" (behaviors) are interrelated and together can exert a positive influence on well-being.

Practical Spirituality is an integrated perspective that focuses on the whole person: mind, body, spirit, family, and community. It views the patient's condition systemically, as all levels from the cellular to the larger group are interconnected. While the medical profession focuses on curing disease, a spiritual perspective puts the person, rather than the illness, at the center.

I embrace a holistic perspective because illness frequently has biological, psychological, and spiritual components. For example, conditions such as high blood pressure, fibromyalgia, digestive difficulties, and headaches, are impacted by emotional states[2] and are correlated with anxiety and depression. Studies show that more than half of patients' visits to doctors' offices are related to psychosocial stressors.[3] That said, a strictly medical model alone is insufficient to address all of these dimensions.

> *"It is a grievous mistake to keep a wall of separation between medicine and religion. There is a division of labor but a unity of spirit…"*
>
> Rabbi Abraham Joshua Heschel

Practical Spirituality values the role spirituality can play in the healing process. I believe it is important for patients to be able to speak not only about their symptoms, but about self, emotions, their families, and relationships. Not only does that clarify the nature of their illness, but it helps them feel more fully understood. We all know that when one person is ill, others are impacted, so care of the patient requires attention to family members as well.

Scientific research demonstrates that our bodies, brains, emotions, beliefs, and even relationships are interconnected and affect one another.[4, 5] For example, having an optimistic mindset may lead people to engage in less-risky behaviors and have a more "can-do" attitude.[6] The placebo effect demonstrates that changes in health can be caused by emotional or symbolic aspects of the healing context.[7] By contrast, "nocebos," such as a noisy, crowded hospital, unfriendly staff, frightening treatments, pessimism, and lack of family support, can increase stress and negatively influence healing.

Practical Spirituality is also a behavioral practice offering a repertoire of spiritual tools to reduce distress and strengthen a patient's sense of perceived coping and control. Practical spiritual tools benefited me by channeling anxiety into constructive activity.

Feeling more in control reduced my distress and increased my persistence in coping efforts. While these tools didn't cure illness, they operated as countermeasures to sustain my spirits. Of course, setbacks in one's condition remind us that much is out of our control as human beings, and we need to rely on powerful others, such as doctors, and ultimately God.

> *"There are two ways to experience life. One is as though nothing is a miracle; the other is as though everything is."*
> Albert Einstein

Just as food is nourishment for the body, I think of spirituality as nourishment for the soul. While spirituality today is widely discussed, it is a perhaps less well-defined phenomenon. I have a sense of the spiritual when I feel awe, such as seeing a rainbow in nature or experiencing the birth of a child.

Awe is defined as a sense of reverence for the mystery of life that transcends rational comprehension,[8] or a sacred sense of the whole that inspires humility.[9] I also find spirituality in moving prayer or when I feel deep gratitude for blessings. Still others experience spirituality through connection with other human beings in fellowship or in a religious community.

Spirituality is broader than religion, which has a more formal language, includes inner faith, rituals, and personal behavioral practices. While people vary greatly in their relationship to spirituality, faith, and religion, surveys show that the majority of Americans feel religion is important in their lives.[10, 11]

Patients surveyed wanted their helpers to be open to religious/spiritual conversations, preferring a holistic approach to their medical care.[12] Patients don't mind if their physician isn't personally religious, but do mind if the doctor is not interested in the patient's spiritual needs.

Even if you are not religious you may be highly spiritual and access spirituality through varied secular pathways such as nature and art. Psychotherapy patients also prefer their practitioners to be open to spiritual matters.[13] While the therapy field has historically been dominated by secular thinking, recently more interest, tools, and training in spirituality have become available.[14, 15, 16, 17]

Can Practical Spirituality and Religion Help a Person Facing Illness?

The answer is a resounding "YES!" Hundreds of research studies show the positive effect of religion and spirituality on patients' lives, making it the "forgotten factor" in physical and mental health.[18, 19] Spirituality is also an ingredient found in long-term satisfying relationships.[20] Numerous writers have identified a "faith factor" in healing from illness,[21, 22, 23] and spiritual practices are linked to resilience.[24, 25] Patients who made remarkable recoveries when diagnosed with terminal illness identified faith as a significant element in their recoveries.[26]

An experienced social work colleague who treats cancer patients, told me that her most fearful patients are those lacking a spiritual side.[27]

Religion and spirituality contain messages than can boost a patient's hope and sense of inner peace, states that positively affect quality of life. Hope is especially important when facing difficult odds.[28] Setting small goals helped me break the spiritual gridlock of passivity, fear, and despair, and move in a constructive direction.

I know a woman who, when pregnant, was struck with breast cancer. Naming her unborn future child "rainbow" encouraged her to weather the illness storm around her. While it is true that hope gets continually redefined as the patient's condition shifts for better or worse, I believe that even terminally ill patients can exemplify hope by finding meaningful time-limited goals.

> *"The tragedy of life lies not in failing to reach our goals,*
> *but having no hope, and thus no goals to reach."*
> Dr. Henry Viscardi, National Center for Disability Services

The root of the word "religion" suggests binding or connecting. The communal aspect of religion provides social support that can reduce the impact of stress. People seem to fare better when connected, and friendships can help us live better, fuller lives. For me, having active spiritual connections broke down the isolation and loneliness experienced during illness.

> *"It is not good for (man) human beings to be alone."*
> Genesis 2:18

Support groups that offer information, validation, and coping skills[29, 30] can lift patients' moods, self-esteem, and confidence by teaching self-regulatory techniques such as meditation. Attending a weekly meditation support group during my treatment and recovery introduced an island of calm into my life.

Participants in multifamily discussion groups are able to share constructive coping strategies, provide mutual comfort, and offer companionship.[31, 32] Support groups, including online groups, can offer significant psychological benefit to enhance quality of life, whether or not life is prolonged.[33, 34]

I am concerned, however, about support groups that mostly vent negative emotions, because they can create anxiety, demoralization, and turn off prospective members.

The spiritually-oriented discussion groups I co-led for patients facing serious medical illness offered a spiritual perspective, spiritual coping tools, emotional support, and community caring.[35] The sessions included soothing music, meditative breathing to calm anxiety, sharing of emotions, creative expression, and discussion of texts to glean traditional Jewish insights. The supportive environment inspired and calmed participants during their difficult time.

The importance of connection and community is illustrated in a beautiful story recounted by Rabbi Harold Kushner, entitled *The Power of Holding Hands.*[36] In it, Kushner describes sitting and watching two children on a beach as they built an elaborate sand castle near the water's edge. Suddenly, despite the careful hard work by the children, a big wave came along, knocked it down, and washed it away. Surprisingly, instead of being devastated, the children ran up the beach laughing and holding hands, and then began building another castle. Kushner concludes that many of the structures we build in life are like on sand, and get knocked down. Only our relationships with others with whom we hold hands will help us endure.

"Practical Spirituality" and Healing

Despite the growing popularity of spirituality in Western culture, the term "healing" is still viewed by some as eerie, non-researched, New Age practices. Healers and shamans, however, existed for millennia in pre-industrial cultures. To the ancients, symptoms were signs of something missing or out of balance in the individual's life or relationships,[37] and healing involved reconnecting to nature, members of the tribe, or the cosmos. Even today, many echo the notion that illness may be a form of disharmony and disconnection, and the purpose of healing is to bring us in harmony with ourselves.[38]

Healing (from the word "*holos*") comes from the same root as whole and holiness, and is about "making whole." Likewise, the Hebrew term "*shelaymut*," (wholeness) is about more than cure or recovery; it is about attaining greater wholeness. For me, healing became about filling the hole in my soul created by illness. While healing can be attained through many pathways, I began renewing and strengthening my spirit by paying attention to my intuition and emotions as a guide.

My definition of healing is quite broad:

- Providing comfort and care to decrease anxiety and suffering.
- Sharing burden to reduce isolation.
- Offering a network of supportive resources.

Healing can include spiritual inspiration from moments of awe, meaningful reconnection to community, finding new purpose, and developing coping skills and strengths. Healing can mean changing one's relationships to self, family, community, and God. Sometimes healing may even involve ending a relationship in the case of a toxic connection. According to Miriam Greenspan, full healing requires one to release the memory of pain from the mind, body, and soul.[39]

> *"Fixing and helping are the basis of curing, but not of healing."*
> Dr. Rachel Naomi Remen

Healing is different from curing. Patients can sometimes attain healing even in the absence of a cure, when they are able to grow spiritually. For example, I believe that my father found healing, despite the continued progression of his serious cardiac illness. In situations of terminal illness, healing may be attained through reconciling interpersonal conflicts with loved ones, achieving a sense of inner peace, or finding closure and comfort during remaining time in life.

Dr. Rachel Naomi Remen uses the term "healing unto death" to describe a person who experiences healing in the process of dying.[40] For example, in the 1990s, the Bay Area Jewish Healing Center in San Francisco offered support groups that created a caring and accepting community for sick, distressed, disabled, and dying AIDS patients. These groups helped patients share burden, explore their spirituality, repair relationships, and strengthen coping skills.

Remen, a chronic illness patient herself, distinguishes between "fixing and helping" and "healing."[41] While helping involves evaluation and judgment, "serving" and "healing" are the work of the soul. Remen wants helpers to recognize the inner wholeness and holiness of each person and themselves. She urges professionals to treat patients as capable partners in the healing process by listening deeply, inviting emotional expression, and showing empathy.

"We serve life because it is holy."

Mother Theresa

Religiously or spiritually-inclined physicians acknowledge their partnership with God in healing. Some doctors pray for inspiration and steadiness in their interventions, and some even pray with their patients or recite prayers on each patient's behalf. I composed a "Healer's Prayer" that I use for personal strengthening, especially after a difficult clinical session with patients. It helps restore me and remind me to be humble, by recognizing the true source of healing for which I am just a conduit.

A Healer's Prayer

Dear God, Source of light and healing,

Thank you for entrusting me with the task of promoting healing and the opportunity to help people.

Help me to open my heart with compassion. Grant me vision and wisdom to guide my patients as they struggle with dilemmas in their lives. Give me strength to challenge my patients to take new steps of growth.

Please protect me with your healing love so that I remain healthy in face of the pain and suffering to which I am exposed. Help me to share, and then release, burdens and responsibilities that are not mine, as I serve as a witness to your healing power.

by Israela Meyerstein

The Patient Nose: A Personal Healing Story

In my mid-forties I was diagnosed with a large skin cancer on my nose that required more extensive surgery than anticipated.

After the operation, I felt ignored and abandoned when the surgeon was nonresponsive and dismissed my questions as irrelevant, preferring to just schedule the next surgery.

> *"Each patient carries his own doctor inside him ... we are at our best when we give the doctor who resides within each patient a chance to go to work."*
>
> Albert Schweitzer

Triggered by a terrifying dream in which I was being chased by a man wielding a knife, some inner spark told me to say "no" to the second surgery, thus beginning my personal healing journey.

> *"Healing proceeds from the depths to the heights."*
>
> Carl Jung

I consulted my inner spirit for guidance to act on my own behalf. I found a new supportive doctor who responded to my questions and respected me. I gave myself permission to make my own health care choices about my nose; after all, it was *my* nose. I found a homeopath who helped me embark on a project of nutritional cleansing, examining confining habits, and embracing positive coping tools such as exercise, visualizations, and affirmations.

> *"A doctor does more by the moral effect of his presence on the patient and family than anything else."*
>
> William James

Strengthened by support from a "village" of friends and new doctors who collaborated with me, I faced the upcoming surgery with more confidence. When the surgeon took another biopsy as I had requested, he found no cancer. Overwhelmed with emotion, I felt truly graced by God. This non-rational transformative moment touched me deeply and opened my eyes to the mysterious process of healing.

I felt inspired and grew spiritually as a result of this peak experience. It led me to co-create and lead spiritual study/ discussion groups to provide support to people struggling with illness. I felt all patients could benefit by learning about spiritual coping tools. In the process, my own spiritual repertoire was strengthened. Little did I know at the time how useful this would soon become in my life.

Looking back, this little cancer was just a "blip on the screen" compared to what came next, which was more than I could have ever imagined. The word "cancer" evokes fear and terror in those diagnosed and in the worried well. You will soon read about my experience facing diagnosis, illness, and the treatment labyrinth. While a very distressing time in my life, my illness journey became a theatre in which I applied down-to-earth spiritual coping tools as countermeasures that strengthened my coping and renewed my spirit. It is my hope that these tools will be useful to you or a loved one facing illness or injury.

Things To Think About And Do

1. Where do you see yourself on a continuum of religion and spirituality?

   *Not at all*_____|_____|_____|_____*Very much*

2. What is your definition of spirituality?

3. Reflect on a time in your life when you experienced awe. What was that like for you?

4. What are your beliefs about a higher power?

5. What does "healing" mean to you?

6. Do you have certain religious or spiritual practices in your life?

7. Is there something missing, disconnected, or out of balance in your life?

8. Is there something you wish or pray for?

Chapter Two
Insights From A Jewish Perspective

Judaism's integrated approach to mind, body, and spirit is evident in the Hebrew language itself. For example, the word *"neshima"* refers to physical breath and *"neshama"* refers to spirit. When we wish someone a *"refuah shelaymah"* it refers to a complete healing of body and spirit. In Judaism, healing is about restoring something within the person that has become lost or hidden from conscious awareness, and less on fixing the person. This strength-based philosophy assumes that the patient can regain wholeness. Just as prisoners cannot free themselves from prison, we cannot heal by ourselves alone because we need each other. The healing triangle consists of the patient, the doctor, and God.[1]

> *"The act of healing is the highest form of 'Imitatio Dei' because God's chief commandment is 'choose life.' The doctor is God's partner in the struggle between life and death."*
>
> Deuteronomy 30:19
> Rabbi Abraham Joshua Heschel

Biblical stories of healing begin with Abraham being visited in his tent by three angels,[2] and his praying to God for Sarah's fertility. When Moses' sister Miriam was struck by leprosy, Moses uttered the first recorded personal prayer in the Bible: "*El na refa na la* – Please God, heal her, please."[3] As a patient, Miriam had to be separated from the community to recover from leprosy, but her healing involved reconnecting to the caring people that would not continue their journey without her.

Later in the *Tanakh* Elisha the prophet is called to a lifeless child's bedside.[4] By the laying on of hands and what resembled CPR, he breathed life back into the child. These early Biblical examples show that human contact is integral to physical and spiritual healing. In a sense, these Biblical healers were precursors to the field of pastoral care that is concerned with the emotional and spiritual needs of the ill.

The awareness that human contact provides emotional comfort explains Judaism's strong emphasis on visiting the sick. A famous Talmudic story of the visit between Rabbi Eliezer and Rabbi Yochanan illustrates how important "being with" the patient is. After a difficult discussion in which the Rabbis cried together, Rabbi Yochanan said, "Give me your hand." He understood the importance of physical comfort when words were not enough.[5]

The Talmud states that "One who visits the sick takes away 1/60 of the sick person's illness and can relieve some of the patient's suffering."[6] Visiting the sick is viewed as an act of godliness as it is believed that the *Shekhinah* (God's feminine presence) dwells at the head of the sick bed. Accordingly, visitors should know their place and not be intrusive. They should do what is needed to make the patient more comfortable, perhaps reciting a prayer. Additionally, they should be sensitive to the severity of the patient's condition, energy level, and tolerance for conversation.

Later Rabbinic codes offer guidelines for when to visit, what to do, where to sit, and what to say. For example, a visitor should sit in front of, but no higher than the patient, and not on the bed. A visitor should discuss affairs of life, not things that promote fear of death. Hospital visits should offer comfort, reduce anxiety, and encourage the patient. With that goal in mind, a colleague and I developed a protocol for using spiritual tools to enhance brief hospital visits. We created a peaceful mood through music, helped patients put their prayerful aspirations into words, and facilitated a feeling of connection to a higher power or people in their community.[7]

Maimonides, a prominent 12th century philosopher and physician, foreshadowed alternative medicine in his emphasis on healthy lifestyle and leading a balanced life. He urged responsible care for our bodies through self-regulation, and viewed moderation in behavior and appetite as keys to a rewarding life. He advocated treating the whole person – body and spirit – and combining spiritual and physiological therapies, believing that the ability to heal from illness depended on giving our bodies the right conditions and atmosphere to heal.

Another significant voice in Jewish healing tradition is Reb Nachman of Breslov (1772-1810). He was referred to as the "tormented master"[8] because of his lifelong struggles with physical illness and depression. He relied on religious faith, cognitive reason, and positive will to combat depression. Reb Nachman's "*Tikkun Klali*," or "comprehensive remedy" for general healing consisted of a specific group of varied Psalms that he felt would uplift the mind, rectify one's failures, and cleanse the soul.[9]

Reb Nachman is also known for his famous inspirational saying:

> "*Kol haolam kulo gesher tzar meod; ve'ha-eekar lo le'fached klal – A person walks in life on a very narrow bridge. The most important thing is not to be afraid.*"

We are all suspended on the bridge of life over troubled waters. While it is hard not to be frightened when ill, I believe his words meant not to succumb to chronic fear, which can paralyze and lead to despair.

Having a purpose elevates our lives spiritually and may even lengthen our years.[10] Some patients positively redefine illness as an opportunity to develop greater appreciation for the blessings and sacredness of life. Illness often teaches us to use our time more wisely.

> *Number our days so as to acquire a heart of wisdom.*
>
> Psalm 90

Like other religions, Judaism recognizes our capacity to grow and repair ourselves and our relationships, as well as pursue self and societal improvement. Eastern religions also emphasize the human's task of continuing Karmic self-improvement until completing one's tasks on earth.

Judaism, a practical and practice–oriented religious and cultural tradition, encourages daily ritual behaviors, faith, and the importance of community connection. The purpose of religious practices is to cultivate spiritual sensitivity and motivate us to perform compassionate deeds in the real world. When we try to repair the brokenness in the world (*tikkun olam*) we reflect our Divine sparks as partners with God.

Things To Think About And Do

1.   How might Maimonides' philosophy of moderation apply to your life?

2.   Visiting a sick patient can remove 1/60 of the illness; is there a friend or person you would like to visit?

3.   Is there something you need healing for?

4.   What would you do to "number your days wisely?"

5.   What might you do to repair the world?

Chapter Three

M.A.P.S. For The Illness Journey

Ｈow do we begin to regain our balance after illness knocks us down and unexpectedly derails us from our life journey? How do we pick ourselves up and search for answers, solutions, and ways to cope? Illness is a disorienting time and patients could benefit by having a map for the territory. My map gave me greater clarity and direction at a time when it would have been easy to succumb to "brain fog," a term often used by cancer patients undergoing chemotherapy. I hope sharing the "M.A.P.S." that helped me on my illness journey will similarly benefit you or a loved one.

I took inspiration from George Albee, a visionary psychologist who developed an elegantly simple but profound "preventive equation"[1] that described how dysfunction occurs. He believed that dysfunction emerges when prevailing stressors and constitutional vulnerabilities (numerator) overwhelm available supports, self-esteem, and coping skills (denominator). If we can develop coping skills that bolster our supportive resources, we can counterbalance the challenges we face and increase our chances of overcoming them. My M.A.P.S. perspective is an outgrowth of this philosophy.

M.A.P.S. is an acronym for **M**eaning or purpose; **A**gency or self-advocacy and empowerment; **P**ractical Coping Tools; and **S**piritual connections. Let me explain.

Meaning

Illness may lack rhyme or reason yet it stimulates searching for answers. While we may never discover an underlying meaning of our illness, constructing meaning by finding new purpose and setting small goals will help us get out of bed each day, give us a sense of coherence, and create a hopeful future orientation. For example, willfully visualizing a future together with his wife helped psychologist Viktor Frankl endure the ordeal of Auschwitz concentration camp during the Holocaust. Frankl later developed a psychotherapeutic approach that encourages people to find their unique task or song, and keep their dignity and sense of hope in order to transcend even the most desperate circumstances.

Agency

Agency refers to being your own representative, with an internal feeling of empowerment and strength, and a belief that you have choices. For me, paying attention to my intuition and trusting my gut emotions helped me feel more self-directed. It further enabled me to become a better advocate for myself in the medical system. Taking active steps further enhanced my sense of agency. Psychologists confirm that a sense of agency is associated with esteem, self-confidence, and adjustment.[2]

Practical Coping Tools

Practical spiritual tools can channel anxiety into constructive activity, give us wider options, and increase our sense of perceived coping. I will describe the wide variety of coping tools I used that are found in complementary and alternative medicine (acupuncture, homeopathy, massage, yoga); creative expression (art, humor, music, poetry); inspirational wisdom, meditative approaches (mindfulness, visualization, guided imagery); nature, prayer, Psalms, stories, texts, and social action that could be potential resources for you.

Spiritual tools do not "cure" illness, but their amazing wisdom is that they provide psychological benefit to the individual who uses them by serving as "countermeasures" to reduce distress and make a difference in how illness or injury is endured. For example, the words and content of prayer can be calming, comforting, and inspiring. They can distract from pain and remind us of blessings, while the patient's active use of prayer can be an antidote to passivity and helplessness that, in turn, leads to persistence in coping efforts.

Spiritual Connections

Spiritual Connections: Being connected helps people feel involved, inspired, cared for, and less alone. Psychologists have found that "communion" or connection is associated with reduced loneliness and greater interpersonal satisfaction.[3] Abundant research shows that social support and connections act as a buffer to illness,[4, 5, 6] and benefit health. When we reach for, receive, and even give social support to others, protective hormones are released in us that stimulate resilience.[7]

A spiritual perspective seeks meaningful connections in life, whether to God, other people, or community. The connection can be internal, to one's inner spirit or Divine spark, or to pathways of creative expression. It can be vertical, to a transcendent force beyond the self, such as God, a higher power or nature. Alternatively, the connection can be horizontal, to other people, such as a religious community with common values, or to friendship and support groups.

Coping with illness is difficult, but these four elements – Meaning, Agency, Practical tools, and Spiritual connections – are cornerstones to building a more stable base of support for patients during difficult times. Moreover, these tools are not just for illness, but lifestyle practices conducive to a healthy body and spirit.

Things To Think About And Do

1. How is your life balanced between stressors and supports?

2. What spiritual tools and resources do you currently use?

3. Where do you turn to for comfort when facing difficult situations?

4. What support systems do you have to connect with?

5. Reflect on a time when honoring your inner spirit made a positive difference in your life.

6. Are you able to construct some meaning out of your illness situation?

7. How might M.A.P.S. be useful on your illness journey?

PART II
THE ILLNESS JOURNEY

Chapter Four

Stuff Happens In Life

March 2006

How does one notice when life slips out of balance? I wish I had a thermometer that measured "stress temperature" as a warning signal before troubles showed up unexpectedly and caught me by surprise. At fifty-eight, my life seemed full and content as I was nearly finished with menopause. I had a full time private practice counseling couples, families, and individuals, did professional writing, played in a Klezmer band, exercised regularly, and volunteered. My life was stimulating and rewarding, but in retrospect, resembled a too tightly-fitting jigsaw puzzle with insufficient breathing space.

Like many couples, our lives ran at a fast pace. We worked hard, played hard, and traveled frequently. We celebrated the weekly joy and peace of the Sabbath that gave us pause to recharge. My "hands-on" responsibilities were considerably reduced when our children left home. While as adults they provided us with tremendous gratification, as a mother I continued to feel worried and anxious as I watched them struggle with difficult situations and I could no longer help them.

My "internal slave driver" continually pushed me to strive to master new challenges and "do it all." As a good oldest daughter, I upheld family tradition by copying my mother's over-functioning, and following my father's advice: "If you want it done right, do it yourself."

Striving for excellence at work was matched by efforts to function as the perfect hostess at home. Holiday celebrations seduced me into ambitious and lavish entertaining. I relished the compliment: "How do you manage to do it all?"

However, my recipe for stress and anxiety made keeping up with me harder than I realized. Add to this substrate some unexpected serious medical crises, and you have a formula for dysfunction as the upcoming Passover holiday put my stress level over the top.

Why Is This Night Different From All Other Nights?
A Passover Ordeal

April 2006

It was the night of the first Passover Seder in a crowded house filled to the brim with a reunion of my siblings, my grown children, cousins, and friends. Hours of cleaning and cooking for the holiday left me feeling tired yet satisfied with the result. As the Seder ritual began, however, I could listen with only one ear. I kept nervously jumping up to check on my 23-year-old son in an adjoining room, who was bent over and clutching his stomach in pain.

He tried to be stoic, but confessed that he'd never felt pain like this before. Earlier in the day he went responsibly to a gastroenterologist, who ruled out appendicitis in favor of a gastric infection. My son re-contacted the doctor, who discouraged him from going to the ER because "it would be a waste of time." I felt helpless as though facing a dead end with no place to go. How could I just watch my son writhe in pain as we began a multi-day holiday weekend?

My mind flitted back and forth between the Passover narrative, my obligations to feed the many guests, and my son's ordeal. As my niece recited the *Ma Nishtana*, ("The Four Questions"), literally meaning "Why is this night different from all other nights?", I thought about how God commanded the Hebrew slaves to suddenly interrupt their lives and flee Egypt, first marking their doors with blood so the firstborn sons would not be slain as the Angel of Death passed over the land.

As my sister and I exchanged wordless glances, recognizing that history had taught us to be "Appendicitis Detectives," we recalled the death of our parents' first child, a 3½-year-old daughter who died after an emergency appendectomy.

I was feeling helplessly stuck and paralyzed like a deer caught in the headlights, yet I couldn't communicate with my husband who was engrossed in entertaining guests and leading the Seder. However, I realized that remaining frozen was not the answer, nor was passivity or despair, the diet of slaves. I knew I must take matters into my own hands. I stood up as if I was getting off a train at an earlier stop and interrupted the Seder, saying: "Can you all just serve dinner yourselves? We're going to the hospital NOW!"

We left hurriedly in the middle of the night under cover of darkness like our ancient Hebrew ancestors. I interrupted a doctor friend in the middle of his Seder and he contacted the hospital to arrange for the necessary tests. He arrived at the hospital at 1:30 a.m. to read the CT scan showing a tangled and infected appendix that needed to come out immediately. Thankfully, he summoned a surgeon in the nick of time.

I returned home the next dawn, exhausted but filled with relief that the Angel of Death had passed over our Jewish household. I was grateful that I had the courage to question the first doctor's diagnosis and act on my own instincts as an act of agency, empowerment, and advocacy for my son. At a personally meaningful level, I realized why this night was different from all other nights!

More Stuff

April-May 2006

The next evening at the second Seder, while my son was still in the hospital, my 85-year-old father-in-law Ralph looked and felt terrible. Within a week he was diagnosed with acute leukemia and was referred to a famous researcher at a prominent local hospital. At the family consultation the doctor was brutally direct. After a brief exam, she delivered a knockout punch, pronouncing a death sentence of less than three months. We were as shocked and numbed by the news as by her tactlessly delivered message. Overnight my father-in-law changed from a feisty independent 85-year-old to a frail patient. From that point on he lost all hope.

During the ensuing days, I remained at his bedside to minister to him and encourage him to eat. I tried "being there" for him during lunchtime and after work, ignoring my own needs for self-care, and surrendering my protective boundaries. My husband was stretched to his limits. I felt I was carrying my father-in-law, his close lady friend, and my husband as well.

I felt sad and helpless as I watched my father-in-law begin his separation from this world. I recognized from my own mother's death the body language signifying death's imminence. At a brief "rally" one evening just before Ralph entered hospice care, my husband read a beautiful healing letter of appreciation to his father.

My last visit to Ralph was on a Friday evening just before the Sabbath. Although he was barely conscious, he seemed soothed by the melody I sang welcoming the Sabbath. As I left I wanted to say "rest in peace," but realized the meaning of the words and couldn't utter them. Instead I said, "Have a peaceful and restful night. It's OK." That night he died.

The whole process from diagnosis to death took less than three weeks. In accordance with Jewish tradition my husband and I stayed in Ralph's room with his body until the Sabbath ended. It was a surreal experience as we spent the day reading Psalms, crying, and recalling incidents from Ralph's life.

At the funeral our sons beautifully eulogized their grandfather, who had been their longest living grandparent. I grieved because Ralph had treated me like a daughter, especially after the deaths of my parents.

During "shiva" (Jewish mourning period) my husband was comforted by the many visitors who came to console him and pray with us. When asked if he had any siblings to support him, my husband answered, "I'm an only child, but at least I have my wife; she will sustain me."

My Turn

June 2006

Following Ralph's death, instead of getting a reprieve after the stressful months, it became my turn. Immediately after shiva ended, I made an appointment with my gynecologist to discuss symptoms that had been troubling me for several weeks. At my recent internal exam I had been pronounced "fine", but shortly thereafter I noticed some occasional, very light pinkish staining along with strange "pieces of tissue." I had to convince the reluctant nurse not to assume it was a urinary tract infection, but instead to take a urine culture. The results showed red and white blood cells, and that test led to a biopsy.

My gynecologist's brief call saying: "The biopsy looks bad. Everything needs to come out. We must get you into surgery as soon as possible" suddenly transported me on an express train to the land of the sick. The doctor saw me the next day together with a gynecological oncological surgeon who would co-perform the surgery and check lymph nodes outside the organs.

To my physician, the focus was on immediately removing offending organs and testing for spread of disease. My concerns were broader: Suddenly my female organs would be gone forever along with a chunk of my identity. I would be out of commission from work for a bunch of weeks and I was facing a lot of uncertainty: How to accept this life-altering change? Worse than that, what if the cancer had spread?

Illness strikes suddenly and catches us unprepared. My scary diagnosis requiring immediate action without time for questions or multiple opinions threw me into confusion and fear. I always assumed I would never rush into major procedures without soliciting multiple opinions, but my doctor's tone of urgency and my trust in him convinced me to move forward immediately. I felt so frightened and desperately searched for something concrete to focus on to help me face this major health and emotional crisis in my life.

I began journaling, a tool I often recommend to patients facing difficult situations. Journaling helped me address my vulnerable feelings of sudden loss and change. A moment before, I was a woman gracefully approaching menopause. The next moment, I was fighting a potentially life-threatening aggressive cancer. In my upset, I sat down and actually wrote an ode personalizing my relationship with my uterus. On the day of surgery I handed my doctor a copy of my musings because I wanted him to understand my emotional and spiritual state. As he read my words, he nodded with gentle amusement, and reassured me that I would be fine.

Diary Of A Uterus At Twilight

June 11, 2006

I am nearly fifty-eight years old. I have served in many ways over the years: helping Israela to feel fully female, carrying and delivering her three fabulous sons, following a regular ebb and flow of the menstrual calendar to lend predictability to her life. Overall, I have done a great job for which Israela is grateful.

In recent years I have been acting up a bit: becoming less predictable, overdoing the bleeding, and creating anxiety and worry in Israela and her doctor. I am grateful for having been allowed to age naturally to help Israela adjust gracefully to her changing life stage. Unfortunately, I have gotten in trouble recently and started to cause trouble as well. I am no longer an organ with a purpose that can contribute anything positive. Israela will be much better off without me. There is no choice; it's time to go.

I am no longer needed for child bearing as Israela is done with raising babies and children. Besides, grandmothers-to-be don't need uteruses. They need a healthy body, strong pairs of hands, and lots of energy to enjoy future grandchildren. In this new life stage it is time for others to bear babies.

I am glad that I have been appreciated and medically well-supervised over the years. May God grant my doctor and surgeon steady hands and clear vision as they remove me. May Israela be blessed with a smooth and steady recovery, renewed vigor, and many years of good health. Amen.

June 12, 2006

Journaling helped me address feelings about my suddenly changing situation. The writing provided a meaningful transitional ritual from one stage to another. On the day of surgery as I lay on the gurney just before my operation, flanked by my interfaith team of doctors including my Jewish gynecologist, Moslem gynecological surgeon, and Christian anesthesiologist, I took out a prayer I had brought with me and read it to bless the doctors' work and pray for a positive outcome.

Mi Sheberach Prayer For Health Care Professionals[1]

For You To Offer

May the One who blessed our Matriarchs and Patriarchs
Sarah, Rebecca, Rachel, and Leah
Abraham, Isaac, and Jacob
bless and strengthen
my doctors
and all who seek to heal those who are suffering.

Imbue them with courage, confidence,
understanding, and compassion
so they may join You
in the work of healing.

May they not surrender in despair,
uncertainty, or fatigue,
but engage in Your work
with wholeheartedness and devotion.
Help them to accompany me
throughout my journey –
to speak with me,
to listen to me,
to be with me
so that together we may strive
for a complete healing,
a healing of body and a healing of spirit,
soon, speedily, without delay,
and let us say,
Amen.

Adaptation of the translation by
Rabbi Simkha Y. Weintraub, LCSW

Although my voice trembled while reading the words from my gurney, my doctors listened attentively, smiled, and nodded "Amen."

This act of agency helped me feel ready for the operation and in the hands of a good collaborative team. My 23-year-old son who was soon to start medical school, stood by my side holding my hand the entire time, reinforcing my belief that he would become a wonderfully sensitive doctor. At the foot of the bed my gynecologist massaged my toes, and it felt wonderful to be touched.

To further calm myself I hummed a Hebrew prayer that encourages relying on God's protection during induced "sleep" (anesthesia) and gentle reawakening.

Adon Olam

Beyado afkeed ruchi be'ayt eeshan ve-ah-eerah – Into God's hand I entrust my spirit, at the time when I am sleeping and when I am awake. Ve'eem ruchi gehveeyahti, Adonai lee v'loh eera. – And with my spirit, I also entrust my body, God is with me, and I will not fear.

Morning Liturgy, Siddur

Until the moment I went under I felt I was actively collaborating with my medical team as a partner in my healing, with caring doctors who were responsive to my needs. Feeling the love and support of my husband, sons, and healthcare team put my body in the best possible shape for surgery and recovery.

The Helper Needs Help

June 13, 2006

The surgeons did their job, stitched me up neatly, and predicted "you'll be fine." Even though I had not yet received the final pathology results, I clung to these words of reassurance. I hugged my silky "*El na refa na la*" healing pillow for comfort, and I pressed the pillow against my abdomen for support as I took my first walking steps in the hospital.

Following major surgery I was forced to rest. My professional life came to an abrupt halt as resting became the order of the day. Although I was tired, limited physically, and unable to perform certain tasks, I never envisioned such a long hiatus from work. I had always conducted my professional practice without interruption, except for maternity breaks, vacations, or minor medical procedures.

As a helper who helped others, suddenly I needed help! I struggled with accepting my new role. No longer the little engine that could," I now became "the little engine that couldn't." Moving from an active doer to a passive recipient was a huge shift. Although I felt uncomfortable accepting help, it was a lesson I needed to learn.

I knew that Jewish tradition strongly mandates a person to accept help when it is truly needed.[2] Friends and family encouraged me to accept offers graciously by pointing out that it would benefit the helpers. I went along, vowing that I would not take advantage of kindnesses.

I contacted clients to offer backup referrals and was touched by their understanding, compassion, and genuine concern, leading me to experience a deeper level of intimacy with them. Being on the receiving end of such warm regard felt nurturing. Additionally, I observed my clients assuming more responsibility for their own lives.

My recovery helped me appreciate the complexities of the healing process, truths I may have known cognitively, but now experienced first-hand: Healing is slow and bumpy, cannot be rushed, happens from the inside out, and requires patience. My own healing process also increased my compassion for my clients' struggles with change.

I carefully followed directions by resting and doing gentle daily exercise to gradually regain my strength and return to work part-time. At my follow up visit, the gynecologist told me I was healing nicely and my lymph nodes were clean. I was ready to put the whole matter to rest. Recovery had seemed simple and straightforward. However, in life, nothing is simple.

Waiting for pathology results that seemed to take forever and were so confounding they had to be sent to Harvard Medical School for evaluation was worrisome. Learning that there were no researched treatment guidelines or even case study data about this very rare cancer occurring only once in 300,000 patients, was even more disconcerting. But an x-ray showing two lung nodules requiring an immediate PET/CT Scan was downright terrifying!

I like feeling special, but this kind of "specialness" was

unwelcome. Because the cancer had invaded the outer layer of the myometrium and was characterized by undifferentiated aggressive cells typically found in the ovaries, my doctor was concerned about recurrence to the lungs or abdomen. He recommended six weeks of prophylactic radiation. Suddenly the "you'll be fine" sounded hollow, as if from far away and long ago. The words were now replaced with new-found worry and uncertainty as I felt myself re-entering the land of the sick.

Things To Think About And Do

1. Journal about your feelings in a diary.

2. Recite a prayer for and/or with your doctor or health care professional.

3. Learn to rest and accept help.

4. Get consultations to increase your options.

5. Try to remember coping skills you used previously when feeling stuck.

6. What comforting messages does your religious or spiritual tradition offer?

7. Reflect on personal habits or tendencies that might need changing.

Chapter Five

The Emotional Landscape Of Patienthood

Apparently the terrorist named "Illness" that kidnapped me planned to keep me for quite a while. The unsettling long-awaited pathology results made it clear that I was embarking on a journey that was unfamiliar even to doctors. I felt I was crossing an invisible border … into an existential territory distinct from the land of the well, a land where others only visit, but at the end of the day, I, the patient, am stuck with the illness.

A young female friend wrote this poignant poem after receiving the shocking news of her Stage 4 Hodgkin's Lymphoma diagnosis.

In An Instant

In an instant, your world can drastically change.

All preconceived notions and expectations can be shattered within seconds.

One day, you can be living your trite, routine life.

You can be partying with friends and adjusting to the nuances of big city life.

Then, in an instant, that all changes.

You receive news that puts life in a new perspective.

You start to appreciate the value of family and friends and shiver at the thought of being without them.

You see beauty in what you used to consider mundane.

And the opportunity to return to a normal life not only seems appealing, but a goal to strive for.

Sometimes, it takes only one instant to gain that perspective.

And hopefully with time, even the most boring days will seem perfect after overcoming the hurdle that simply took an instant of time.

Rachel Minkove, November 2008

The illness experience is broader than the disease and shatters our basic assumptions of invulnerability. It is a difficult journey because of the emotional baggage that comes along on the trip: a suitcase of difficult feelings such as fear, anger, sadness, confusion, guilt, and despair; spiritual questions without answers, such as "why me?" and "what did I do to deserve this?" and a passport to the sick track.

As I entered the unfamiliar territory of the hospital environment I had to undergo numerous procedures and anxiously wait for results communicated in complex medical terms for which I had no experience interpreting. The climate of uncertainty undermined my self-confidence and problem solving. I could see that sustaining my spirits and preserving identity would be a challenging endeavor.

Not only are patients trapped in this new territory, but ripple effects spread to family members, who have their own emotional reactions to diagnosis and prognosis, and may feel helpless watching their loved ones suffer. Some family members suppress their feelings to protect the patient, a common phenomenon among men whose wives have breast cancer,[1] and some patients hide their feelings in order to avoid upsetting family members.

Having family members present at doctor's appointments is helpful because patients often don't retain much of the information given by the doctor. The presence of a family member caregiver also alters the balance of power and may give the patient more courage to speak up.[2]

Family members often have no preparation before they are thrust into the caregiver role. Because of the demands of the job they may ignore their own emotional stress and health out of a sense of responsibility for the patient. Caregivers, while often the healthier family members, are devotedly committed to helping, but may be like the shoeless kids of the cobbler whose needs go unnoticed. Caregivers could also benefit from support and expressive outlets to lower their distress.

I recall many years ago that it was so hard for me to find support as a family member when my mother was dying of pancreatic cancer in 1981 at a famous New York hospital. Overwhelmed, I begged to speak with someone who could "help us cope." However, no social worker showed up during the nine months between my mother's diagnosis and death. I was horrified that one arrived only a few hours before my mother's death to tell us the obvious: that she would soon die.

I observed my father's growing sadness and terror as a caregiver and a physician who fully understood the prognosis. He was a spiritual but non-religious person, yet curiously, as he faced my mother's terminal illness, even he sought help from a higher power.

I Am Sad Today

© George Gorin, 1980.

I am sad today,
Gone are the sparkles in her eyes;
Where are the blue fountains?

I am sad today,
Shadows of despair
Darkened her eyes.

I am sad today,
Her smile froze
On her face.

I murmur a prayer to my God:

Please revoke the verdict
If not for my sake,
Please do it for Her.

Despite facing a terminal illness, my mother put on a courageous smile and maintained her strong upbeat stance until the end, probably to protect us. She put her faith in a religious doctor's experimental treatments and remained reluctant to use complementary medicine techniques to improve breathing and comfort. I don't know whether she attained a sense of "healing," but perhaps her faith gave her a sense of peace. As a family we did not have formal conversations about her dying. Only to our apartment neighbor did my mother confide: "I'll see you in another world."

We stayed at my mother's bedside until the end, showering her with love, patting her face with cool water, and pretending a fantasy trip to her favorite beloved seashore. She gave final hugs to me and for the grandchildren, and I held her hand through the last hours until she slipped away. Like a regal queen with her devoted entourage at her side, she had a beautiful death if death can ever be described that way.

My mother's illness and death pushed my father out of his private self to express strong inner emotions and grieving. The following year my father survived his own life-threatening heart surgery, and emerged as a full-time poet. Through poetry, he purged life-long melancholic feelings about the traumatic loss of home and country, the murder of his family during the Holocaust, and the death of his first baby daughter. He shared feelings he had not been able to fully express while my mother was alive. With the help of a new supportive intimate relationship, his spirit visibly lightened and he seemed to get younger emotionally with each passing year as he recovered his lost childhood.

Although my father's cardiac illness continued to progress, his emotional expression expanded in a way that seemed like a spiritual healing. Just before his last surgery, the one he didn't survive, he completed his final book of poetry with a poem in the form of a prayer to his surgeon. On what turned out to be my last visit with him, he asked me to calligraph what he wrote, a task I had lovingly done for him many times over the years.

The Lifeguard

© George Gorin, Life on Edge (1990)

~ *To Frank Spencer, Heart Surgeon* ~

*He roams the shore
of life searching
with an eagle's eye*

for those caught
in a maelstrom: people
drowning, gasping for air

in the turbulence
between life and death.
There isn't much time

when victims grasp
at a straw of hope
while sinking and

resurfacing for a last
look at Mother Earth.
I am praying for a

firm grasp of the
lifeguard's hand
while my whispers
ascend skywards.

Clearly, my father's poetry was his spiritual coping tool. In the trenches of intensive care the year after my mother's death, even he turned upwards towards a higher power. Perhaps as my father's daughter, I inherited his wisdom about creative expression as a pathway to spiritual healing.

The Medical Labyrinth

July 2006

It may seem strange to say that the overwhelming difficulties of illness are merely the tip of the iceberg, but navigating today's high tech medical system can be an unexpected challenge. Patients must absorb complex information, evaluate different medical opinions, and sometimes even be their own case managers. My prior brush with illness provided only the most rudimentary experience.

My doctor prescribed six weeks of prophylactic radiation, so I set up an appointment at the hospital and parked in a "privileged" spot reserved for radiation oncology patients. I had to pinch myself as I entered: *Was this really happening to me?!* I realized that people in the waiting room were cancer patients, but I felt reluctant to accept my new status. How would I get used to this? Would I always have this identity?

July 25, 2006

The chatty Radiation Oncologist talked more about her family issues than my situation, which I found a bit off-putting. She confidently endorsed radiation as the way to go and called my case "routine." Puzzled, but relieved to hear her interpretation, I scheduled appointments for daily radiation for the next six weeks.

Only a few hours later on the very same day I consulted with the head of Medical Oncology at a leading teaching hospital, hoping to receive his endorsement of my treatment plan. After waiting over two hours, the doctor greeted me by extending a limp two-finger handshake, and seated himself at least ten feet away from me as if cancer was contagious. He glanced at my records, consulted with his assistant who had interviewed me, then handed down his dictum.

First, he sharply disagreed with the plan for radiation, stating that the danger of recurrence was 40%, far greater than the 15-25% my surgeon had predicted. He strongly suggested doing chemotherapy first because radiation would destroy veins, making chemotherapy impossible. He criticized my surgeon (who had been his teacher) for taking out only several nodes for testing, stating that he would have removed at least twenty to thirty. His comments undermined confidence in my surgeons' recommendations. Did he realize that demeaning another doctor's work profoundly affected the patient? I felt as if he had pulled out the rug from under me.

Since there were no clinical trials, research, or multiple case studies for the cancer I had, the best he could offer for my cancer was a standard unproven treatment protocol. He gave me literature about chemotherapy, then offered me the same limp hand shake, leaving me no time for processing the information or asking questions. I guess he didn't expect anyone to question him. I thought of Heschel's quote:

"The mother of medicine is not human curiosity, but human compassion, and it is not good for medicine to be an orphan." [3]

I felt quite shaken by this consultation because it undermined my prescribed treatment plan and especially because of his remote style. I couldn't imagine putting myself in his care. I felt like I was a spinning top in the Tower of Babel, confused by different experts' recommendations. I felt frightened wandering through the maze of the medical labyrinth, jostled and jolted from side to side by conflicting opinions. I wanted to depend on some experts, but what do you do when the structure you are leaning on feels like a house of cards?

July 27, 2006

Two days later I met with a medical oncologist at the local community hospital, hoping he would break the tie to end my confusion. The busy doctor fit me in on his last day before vacation. After reviewing my records he warmly shook my hand and spoke directly and persuasively about the need for chemotherapy. "You must do this for your best chances," he said.

He told me that he had personally gone into the lab, inviting two experienced pathologists with him to examine my slides. He was concerned that the cells looked aggressive, undifferentiated, and "angry," and he concurred about the danger of recurrence in the absence of aggressive treatment.

He explained that when clinical trials are unavailable, using standard protocol is not advisable. Rather, he would individualize treatment because each patient is unique and reacts differently to treatment. Moreover, each patient comes with different abilities, strengths, weaknesses, culture, and life experiences. What a novel idea and music to my ears! When he said that "each patient is an individual, not a statistic" I was sold. Statistics give rough outlines, referring to large groups of people, yet can strongly impact a patient's mood and outlook. I felt much more hopeful as an individual than as a statistic.

This doctor fostered confidence by his intelligence, compassion, and innovative thinking. He seemed to be a bit of a maverick and advocated using a more recently-discovered chemical agent that breaks up blood vessel formation. I felt his genuine concern for my welfare as he took time to listen to me and patiently answered my questions. His nurse told me that he is very involved with his patients, often stopping by during their infusion center visits.

Selecting A Doctor

July 28, 2006

> *"The doctor must find out the pressure of the blood and the composition of the urine, but the process of recovery also depends on the pressure of the soul and the composition of the mind."*
>
> Rabbi Abraham Joshua Heschel, 1964

Research confirms that patients yearn to be treated as people, not just another case.[4] They value doctors' personal attributes of compassion, caring, and being a good listener. The word "patient" means "one who suffers," and "compassion" and "sympathy" mean "to suffer with." Patients want respectful, trustworthy, and collaborative partnerships with their physicians.

The origin of the word "medicine" is "mederi," which means paying attention to facilitate well-being. Not surprisingly, the word "cure" is related to the word "care," echoing Francis Peabody's belief that the secret of patient care is caring for the patient.[5]

> *"People will forget what you said, people will forget what you did, but people will never forget how you made them feel."*
>
> Maya Angelou

Despite doctor friends warning me to get treatment only at a National Comprehensive Cancer Center in Baltimore or New

York, I overcame my uncertainty and followed my gut that said "go with this guy." After all, it is my body and therefore my choice and responsibility. Traveling to frequent treatments at the local hospital would be easier on me, so I decided with my heart, which was an act of personal agency. After sending my materials to a third expert, who gave vote #3 for doing chemotherapy first, I scheduled six chemo treatments, once every three weeks over a period of five months, to be followed by six weeks of daily radiation. It seemed like it would be a long period in my life.

"Both And"

August 3, 2006

Walking the fence between Biomedicine and Complementary and Alternative Medicine is a balancing act I have long practiced. The dual process has left me feeling enriched, at times conflicted, and occasionally buoyed when the approaches complement one another. At first, like many patients, I felt apprehensive about telling my biomedical doctors about my alternative practitioners for fear of criticism, but I came to realize how beneficial the exchange of information is to each professional's approach and to the patient.

Over the years I have consulted with a homeopath who treats the whole person in context: body, mind, spirit, and life-style practices. This approach matches my systemic perspective of the patient as an interconnected living system. Before beginning chemotherapy I met with my homeopath, who agreed that a systemic "big guns" approach such as chemo was needed for my condition. He offered me nutritional guidelines, digestive enzymes to maximize absorption, and guidance for the spiritual journey. He emphasized creating a less acidic, more alkaline internal environment, so I began checking my pH daily to get feedback on my internal climate and food choices.

He also asked me to reflect on my life-style and emotional habits, which were as important to him as nutrition and medical treatments. He invited updates from me, and projected working with me after my treatments to strengthen immune system recovery.

Like other cancer patients, I had a treatment entourage

consisting of a large host of helpers: medical oncologist, surgeon, specialists (i.e. gynecologist, urologist, radiation oncologist, radiologist, pathologist, internist, to name a few). Each specialist focused on a different part of the proverbial elephant that is the patient's body.

In my ideal world these multiple helpers from different perspectives would communicate with each other and operate as a collaborative team in viewing the patient as a whole person. Also, many patients could benefit from having a patient coordinator to help them navigate the complex treatment labyrinth. Otherwise patients are left to gather the pieces and assemble the puzzle themselves.

I knew I was embarking on an important program for the next six months of my life that would require a variety of supports. I increased the frequency of acupuncture treatments to help my body deal with the effects of chemo, strengthen my blood, and for general well-being. My acupuncturist offered her presence, patient listening, and genuine concern, as well as nutritional and lifestyle recommendations.

During this period I also integrated several tools from my Jewish tradition, music, and nature to put together a musical mini-prayer service to sing when I sat outside or walked in nature. I sang three prayers to focus my mind and heart on gratitude to God for:

- Allowing me to wake up in the morning (*Modeh Ani*)
- The wondrous design of the human body (*Asher Yatzar*)
- The Divine spark breathed into me (*Elohai Neshama*)

Angels Among Us

In the wilderness of illness, patients at times encounter voices that are like angelic guides for the journey. Some consider angels to be heavenly messengers on earth, offering consolation, comfort, and protection as expressions of God's love for his children. Angels remind us of our connection to the Divine and our potential for holiness through our actions in the world.

While not emphasized in modern Jewish tradition, angels

have played significant roles since recorded Biblical history, and they appear in legends and life cycle rituals, such as the weekly song welcoming the Sabbath. They are also thought to be active and engaged in conception, protecting pregnancy, birthing, and death. A pair of angels is said to accompany each of us everywhere, to prevent loneliness and remind us of our intimate connection with God.[6]

> *"God will instruct His angels to watch over you wherever you go."*
>
> Psalm 91:11, Midrash Psalms 17:8

In Jewish tradition four angels are thought to surround the sick person. On the right side is *Michael* (who is like God, the right hand of God); on the left is *Gavriel* (the strength of God, to overcome fear); in front is *Uriel* (the light of God for clear vision); and behind is *Rephael* (the healing of God). Hovering above and all around them is *Shekhinah*, the feminine healing Presence of God.

In Christianity it is said that when you pray for someone, an angel sits on the shoulder of that person.[7] The Archangel Raphael is considered the heavenly physician in Christianity. My homeopath has a picture of Raphael on his wall above where the patient sits to remind him that healing comes from God. Each morning the doctor asks for Raphael's guidance to make him an instrument of Divine will.

During my illness experience angels came in several forms. First was the caring, concerned voice of a supportive friend, who asked incisive questions at just the right time. Before surgery she emailed me a list of practical tips for dealing with a hysterectomy and hospital stay, such as keeping the doctor's cell phone number at bedside, and bringing a supportive pillow for starting to walk again after surgery.

When my friend saw that I was just numbly following the first treatment plan offered, she encouraged me to seek consultations before moving forward, and gave me the name of a doctor who might help with referrals. I wondered: I am a mental health professional with graduate training; how do poor people with little resources, connections, or insurance evaluate their treatment options and navigate the complex system?

My friend also organized a corps of women to prepare meals for me on chemotherapy days, which felt enormously helpful and comforting. She insistently reminded me to learn to accept help because she knew that caregivers like me seem to have particular difficulty relying on others. How can I describe her except to call her an angel?

Another angel on my journey was an exceptionally kind nurse in the gynecological surgeon's office. At my follow-up visit six weeks after surgery, the nurse took it upon herself to refer me to a medical oncologist who ultimately became my doctor. I had never even heard of that specialty, but came to learn that it describes a doctor who treats cancer systemically.

The nurse was an angel in other ways as well. On that same postoperative visit I reported having a strange cough. Since the likely places the cancer might have spread were the lungs or pelvis, the surgeon immediately recommended a CT scan of the lungs. I was shocked as two lung nodules were found. The nurse understood my panic and arranged a PET/CT scan for me the very next day – on Saturday, the Jewish Sabbath.

Shabbat Morning Prayer At The PET/CT Scan

Having a PET/CT scan was not my usual way of "resting" on the Sabbath, but urgency was of essence. I sat alone in a darkened room for a long while, drinking a tall glass of liquid. Anticipating what the test might find engendered tremendous, almost paralyzing anxiety. I grasped for something to keep me busy and calm my fears while I waited. I turned to the wisdom of Psalms and began reciting – actually singing – Psalm fragments in Hebrew to focus my attention, express my inner emotions, and feel less anxious. Connecting with my Jewish tradition felt strengthening and helped me feel less alone. My efforts resulted in an emotionally powerful spiritual experience.

First, I offered prayers of gratitude for how far I had come in recovering from my surgery:

> *"Modeh ani lefanechah, melech chai vekayam – I thank God, the everlasting King."*
>
> Siddur, Morning Liturgy

I knew that I was in a narrow place of worry and searching for answers. I felt small and powerless and sang a Psalm expressing my yearning:

> *"Min hamaytzar karati ya, anani bamerchavya – From the narrow depths I call to You, O God; please answer me with Your expansiveness."*
>
> Psalm 118; Hallel

I found words of my tradition floating in and out and carrying my feelings along with them. The words seemed so relevant to me at this time of vulnerability.

> *"Nafshi cholah ahavatecha, ana el na refa na la – My soul is ill, with your love, please heal her."*
>
> Piyut Yedid Nefesh, Rabbi Elazar Azhari.
> www.piyut.org.il

I felt very needy, and asked for help, inspiration, and rescue:

> *"Esa eynai el heharim, mei ayin yavo ezri – I lift my eyes to the mountains whence my help shall come."*
>
> Psalm 121

I tried to breathe deeply, imagining oxygen flowing and God's Divine breath circulating throughout my body's cells:

> *"Elohai neshama shenatata bee tehora hee. Atah beratah, atah yetzarta, atah nefakhta bee, v'atah meshamrah bekeerbee. – My God, the soul which You have given me is pure. You created it, You formed it, You breathed it into me. You keep body and soul together."*
>
> Siddur, Morning Liturgy,
> Birkot Hashachar; Berakhot 60b

I felt small and powerless as I breathed, prayed, and acknowledged that I was in God's hands and healing grace. Vulnerable tears of beseeching poured down my face. I thought of the Psalm (13:2) that mentions *"Al Tastir,"* (don't hide your face from me) and sang the beautiful Debbie Friedman melody[8] about it.

I envisioned family ancestors (my mother, father, and aunt), who are no longer here, but who always loved and protected me. Suddenly I sensed a bright light shining on me that induced feelings of awe and disbelief. The words tumbled out of my mouth:

> *"Kadosh, kadosh, kadosh, Adonai tzevaot, mehloh khol haaretz kvodo – Holy, holy, holy, God's luminaries fill the whole world with glory."*
>
> Liturgy, Siddur

I felt my fear convert into budding hope and faith. I tried to remain open and vulnerable:

> *"Kol haneshama tehallel yah – Every living thing that breathes praises You, O God."*
>
> Siddur, Hallel Psalm 145-9

I continued to breathe, imagining golden healing light preparing my cells to undergo the severe scrutiny of the PET/CT scan machine. I was told to lie on the table with my hands stretched over my head, so I held them in a praying clasp. I closed my eyes to focus more internally and not be unnerved by the loud movements of the machine. I worried what the scan would show. An image arose of missiles aimed at the lung nodules, and I began to breathe heavily and with determination through my tears.

I shed more cleansing hopeful tears:

> *"Yehi ratzon imri pi vehegyon leebee lefanecha Adonai tzuri v'goahli – May the words of my mouth and the meditation of my heart be acceptable to You , my God, my rock and my redeemer."*
>
> Liturgy, Siddur

After what seemed like forever, the test was over. Relief was quickly replaced by having to anxiously wait until the next week for results. And then ... a small miracle! The technician asked a radiologist to come in specifically to read the results. Upon returning home, I received a call from my "angel nurse" sharing the results: "normal." More tears, but this time tears of joy:

> *"Hazorim bedeemah bereenah yiktzoru – Those who sow with tears shall reap with joy."*
>
> Psalm 126

In gratitude, I wrote letters of commendation about the technician and nurse for their outstanding care.

It Takes A Village

Because the road to healing is rarely straight and has numerous bumps along the way, it takes a supportive village to care for the patient. I gratefully accepted the care and concern shown to me by knowledgeable professionals, family, friends, and my *chavurah* (friendship community). One very busy friend routinely sent me get well cards to show her caring. Others invited me out to lunch when I was up to it. It made me feel loved and supported while going through my struggle.

However, even receiving support can be a complicated matter. Patients feel differently about sharing personal information about their bodies and providing detailed updates, especially about certain medical conditions, such as gynecological and urological.

Patients and family members may have to act as "gatekeepers" who assess which of the many well-intentioned friends and relatives in the patient's social network are respectful of boundaries and provide useful support, and which wind up draining the patient's energy through excess curiosity and communication. The responsibility for boundary maintenance is yet another job patients must learn, but one that can stimulate healthy agency and self-care.

Things To Think About And Do

1. Have patience with yourself; illness is a lot to deal with.

2. Accept your feelings without judgment; feelings are not good or bad.

3. Ask a family member or friend to come to appointments for lending support and processing information.

4. Check with your gut and inner spirit as a guide in choosing a doctor.

5. Consult with other experts to make wise and thoughtful decisions.

6. Speak up and/or change doctors if you don't feel treated respectfully as a person.

7. Remember that you are an individual, not a statistic.

8. Select creative coping tools to calm your anxiety, lift your spirits, and inspire you.

9. Consider being open to angels and Divine intervention; do *your* angels have names?

10. Gather a village of helpers and allow them to care for you.

Chapter Six
The Strange World Of Dr. Chemo

August 11, 2006 – December 29, 2006

Thank God, oncologists can prescribe many poisons to give us that destroy aggressive cancer cells! I felt encouraged by my doctor's confident manner, but also wary due to the seriousness with which he approached my situation. An orientation session at the Infusion Center helped prepare me for my coming ordeal by describing the various mild to dangerous side effects of chemotherapy. In response to what I heard, I engaged in self-protective denial, because I wanted to continue life as usual and not lose things, especially my hair. Outwardly, I accepted the upcoming regimen but internally I resisted, wanting to hold on to my "normalcy" as long as possible.

Despite being told directly that I would become bald by the second treatment, I kept hoping to be the exception to the rule. For many women the impact of hair loss is greater than the loss of organs, including breasts. Some elect to shave their heads to feel more in control over the process. I rather held on to each last clump of hair, gradually having to cover up with kerchiefs, bangs, and eventually wigs.

Entering the hospital's Infusion Center felt like stepping into a strange world consisting of many cubicles, each with a privacy curtain and furnished with a big easy chair to make the visit as homey and comfortable as possible. To avoid feeling swallowed up into the center I requested a cubicle nearest the window so I could look outside and see a bit of nature. This gesture was part of my desperate attempt to hold on to my quickly fading normalcy.

Outside the center's front door was a lovely rock garden. I brought a magic marker and after each visit I inscribed words on a rock such as "fear," "hope," "gratitude," "new twins." This minor act of documenting signposts along my journey became a way of emotionally acknowledging my experience.

Feeling energetic after my first chemo treatment because I was pumped up with prophylactic steroids, I made a crazy escapist trip to New York City to see a Chihuly exhibit at the Bronx Botanical Gardens with my sisters. I was eager to bond with them, and they with me. Toward the end of the day, however, creeping fatigue, nausea, and exhaustion overcame me, and I realized it was my punishment for pushing the envelope. I quickly learned humility and a healthy respect for powerful chemicals that could control my well-being to a large degree.

It didn't take long for me to discover that chemotherapy was more like a marathon with numerous hurdles to overcome than a sprint. While each session was scheduled to take about four hours, instead six or seven hours were the norm. There was a lot of waiting built in for drawing blood, sending it to the lab, ordering from the pharmacy, and delivery. In addition each nurse routinely treated several patients at the same time.

On my first day of treatment, I was cared for by a somewhat proper nurse with a British accent who explained all the procedures, the sequence and timing of the medicines, and the likely side effects. The first order of business was drawing blood. She presumed I would get a port in my chest to make it easier for the nurses to draw blood, but I didn't want a port because it would prevent me from swimming, one of my favorite exercise and relaxation outlets.

I tried to guide her to likely successful spots for finding a vein, but she insisted on following her own ideas about where to stick me. After her fourth failed attempt, she proclaimed: "My dear, you have feeble veins." I knew my veins were challenging, but neither I nor they appreciated this disparagement. Perhaps this was the moment when my inner spirit decided to create a practical spiritual toolbox to help me survive and cope.

I prepared myself for the next blood drawing by drinking more water. As the nurse began searching for veins, I closed my eyes and sang a special Hebrew prayer describing the Divine creation of the human body with its vessels and channels that must open or close for proper functioning. At once intimate and universal, this blessing recognizes man's fragility and God's providential care.

The prayer is *Asher Yatzar*, recited by traditional Jews each morning after rising and using the toilet. Rather than take our bodily functions for granted, this prayer gratefully acknowledges God's sovereignty and creative power over our biological functioning with awareness of our spiritual nature of being created in the Divine image.

The prayer as translated in English, reads:

> *"Blessed are You, O Lord our God, King of the universe, who has formed man in wisdom, and created in him many orifices and vessels. It is revealed and known before the throne of Your Glory, that if one of these be opened, or blocked, it would be impossible to exist and to stand before You. Blessed are You, O Lord, who heals all flesh and does wondrously."*
>
> Morning Liturgy, Siddur[1]

Singing the Hebrew words and beautiful melody by Debbie Friedman[2] helped me turn inward to access an almost meditative state as I visualized my blood flowing wondrously through my veins. What really made the difference, however, was letting go and acknowledging God's creative power.

When I used this prayer as a coping tool, the nurses' batting average improved from four to five tries down to one or two. I shared the prayer with several nurses who asked for a copy to use with their spiritually-oriented patients. One nurse told me that she said a prayer as well: "O Lord, guide me to those veins."

I approached subsequent chemo sessions with a plan by coming equipped with a "chemo kit" consisting of a CD visualization to use during the different chemo drug administrations, colored pencils and a doodling pad, some light reading material, music, and my soft healing pillow with the words "Please God, heal her please" in Hebrew. I also brought my journal book that has a cover design with flowers and a quote by Thoreau: "Go confidently in the direction of your dreams. Live the life you've imagined." I packed some light snacks in case I had no appetite for the hospital food offered during lunch time.

As I listened to a Belleruth Naparstek CD[3] specifically tailored to enhancing the benefits of chemotherapy, the imagery guided me to visualize a "circle of allies" that joined me in a safe place and helped me feel I had a supportive, protective team. Images of my mother and other caring relatives appeared, even though they are no longer alive. The imagery of white healing light suggested the powerful workings of chemo. The beautiful colors described and Naparstek's soothing voice helped me relax and even doze off.

I learned the names of the drugs (Carboplatin, Avastin, and Abraxane), and during each drug administration I did some

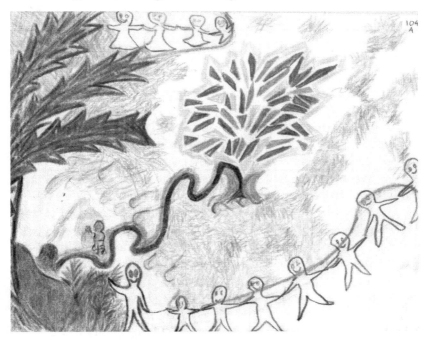

The author's "circle of allies" imagery.

doodling, using my imagination to play with the name of the drug and how it was supposed to work. For example, Avastin targeted tumor blood vessel formation, so I sketched a shooter that blasted little collections of vessels. Abraxane imaginatively became "abracadabraxane," and with a whimsical doodling, I hoped for its magical effects. I found that drawing, an activity I have always loved, distracted me and helped me manage my anxiety during the long chemo sessions.

At times the meds induced sleep. I preferred having my curtain drawn as a shield to avoid having to watch other chemo patients in cubicles opposite me having nauseating reactions. I personally found it easier to be alone, and more taxing to host visitors. I know that other patients appreciate visitors for conversation, and distractions of television, video games, or iPhone apps.

As for company, I didn't want my husband to have to miss work. Besides, making conversation took social energy I didn't have. One time my son came to sit with me, but when I saw how hard it was for him to see me in my condition it was actually easier for me emotionally to let him go so I could retreat into rest. I thanked friends or family who offered to visit, but remained honest and protective of my needs; this certainly wasn't the time to accommodate to what made others comfortable.

And so I whiled away the hours using my creative imagination and my kit of spiritual coping tools. The "countermeasures" calmed my anxiety, gave me something active to do, and bolstered my confidence in my coping abilities. It is important for patients to find their own preferred form of positive distraction that feels supportive and strengthening. Since sessions are a long haul, it is a good idea to come prepared.

The staff of the Infusion Center was largely kind and caring. My mood was bolstered whenever my doctor stopped in to check on me. I learned about available ancillary services, and met with the medical social worker and patient advocate.

I got used to the chemotherapy regimen after one or two cycles, and as predicted, by the second treatment I was completely bald. I had great difficulty with losing my hair, at first slowly, and then quite rapidly. A friend I had appointed to be my humor and laughter coach during treatment sent me a story that lightened my mood and put things in perspective.

Three Hairs

There once was a woman, who woke up one morning,
Looked in the mirror,
And noticed she had only three hairs on her head.
"Well," she said, "I think I'll braid my hair today."

So she did. And She Had A Wonderful Day.
The next day she woke up,
Looked in the mirror
And saw that she had only two hairs on her head.
"H-M-M," she said,
"I think I'll part my hair down the middle today."
So she did. And She Had A Grand Day.

The next day she woke up,
Looked in the mirror and noticed that
She had only one hair on her head.
"Well," she said,
"Today I'm going to wear my hair in a pony tail."
So she did. And She Had A Fun, Fun Day.

The next day she woke up,
Looked in the mirror and noticed that
There wasn't a single hair on her head.
"YEA!" she exclaimed,
"I don't have to fix my hair today!"

Attitude is everything.

Spiritual Parable
Author Unknown

I decided to use my new bald state as an opportunity to experiment with different hair styles, something I hadn't done in many years. I took advantage of the American Cancer Society's free wig service, talked to people about head coverings, and attended "Feel Good Look Better" sessions to get free makeup and support. I was determined to squeeze lemons into lemonade.

I still was hoping to keep the rest of my life the same by continuing to work. Experience taught me that after treatments I would be wiped out for a week like a bad flu, but then I would recover and have two decent weeks before the next treatment. As time went on however, cumulative effects of chemo took their toll, taking over my life even more. While I hoped to prop myself up longer, the pyramid of losses – loss of physical comfort, of predictability and control, and finally – my hair, prevailed.

One day I came down with a virus that completely wiped me out. As chemo progressed, I worried that I might feel this bad more of the time and I questioned whether I could get up each morning to see an office full of patients. Thanks to this little virus bug and a friend's support, I decided to stop working. Continuing to work would have pushed me beyond my limits and left me worn out mentally and physically, and what would that have accomplished?

Consulting my inner spirit, I chose rest instead of work. I was grateful that my economic situation, with my husband's income and my disability coverage, made the decision feasible, but it was not easy to "abandon" my practice, fearing it might result in professional suicide. I made arrangements to refer out patients who needed ongoing treatment. This was the first time in over twenty years of practice that I totally stopped work.

I was touched and heartened by clients' good will and caring prayers. Some stayed in touch but no one violated the boundaries of my rest. When potential new clients called, I took down their contact information for the future. At the time I couldn't focus on the challenge of reviving my practice, but perhaps stating I would return represented hope for the future.

Taking a medical sabbatical allowed me to let go of the heavy and stressful job of supporting people in their lives for which I may have felt too responsible. Emotionally it was hard for me to let go, because I have always prided myself in "being there" for my patients.

The lighter schedule relieved stress and helped me focus on my own healing. I began attending a meditation group at Hopewell Cancer Support in Baltimore.

There my favorite meditation consisted of a long visualized trip to a favorite place, then to a chalet in the field. In the cellar of the chalet I was invited to "take something needed" out of a large chest. Each time I surprised myself by retrieving just what I most needed emotionally, such as patience, hope, appreciation. Receiving the "medicine" I needed positively affected my mood well after the meditation sessions.

My new "under-functioning" position, totally antithetical to me, was just what I needed to do. Being responsible for me first and foremost, and coping with the difficult side effects of treatment was enough of a job. Realizing that I simply lacked the strength to over-function lessened my guilt about stopping work. Besides, a very new joy was on the horizon – twin granddaughters. I wanted to have energy to make special time for them as they entered the world.

I came to view this decision as crucial in making the difference between drowning versus surviving, coping, and even thriving. The gift of rest is the most precious commodity in today's world. I hoped it would allow me to do a lot of personal reflection and become better and wiser for the experience.

I believe that every patient can benefit by developing a down-to-earth practical spiritual toolbox, but it is up to the individual to decide which tools to include that resonate most personally. Some people may prefer turning inward for strengthening, such as through meditation. Others may reach outwards to various distractions, to friends, or to a religious community, and some may choose a combination of all of the above.

Trying to heal from illness or injury is a time to consult one's inner spirit for direction rather than to accommodate to others' wishes and ideas. While all decisions contain risks, focusing on what I, as the patient, needed most, gave me the precious gift of healing from the inside out.

Things To Think About And Do

1. Consult your inner spirit to identify and speak up about your needs.

2. Write an inspirational word on a rock or card for strengthening.

3. Learn about supportive resources for your particular illness.

4. Make use of a patient navigator or coordinator to access needed services.

5. Find a healing visualization to lift your spirit.

6. Assemble a "chemo kit."

7. Take a pillow or comfort object to hold.

8. Listen to music or doodle.

9. Try wigs, makeup, and explore new hairstyles to feel attractive.

10. Give yourself the gift of time to rest.

11. Remember that what works for you, the patient, is the way to go!

Chapter Seven

Radiation: A Less Than Illuminating Experience

December 21, 2006 – February 7, 2007

G rateful that I had weathered chemotherapy fairly well, I prepared to start six weeks of daily radiation. Friends who had undergone radiation downplayed its difficulty, saying: "It's no big deal; you'll just feel a little tired." I took their word for it cautiously, because I knew that no two patients, illnesses, or treatments are alike. I now had an appointment every day of the week for the foreseeable future.

The radiation department, nicknamed "the vault," had a depressing retro feel, and was housed in the basement of the oldest part of the hospital. I wondered if the basement location was needed to contain all the toxic radiation to which I would be exposed. As I entered, the reception staff sent me to the waiting area down the hall without giving any instructions. A fellow patient there pointed out where the gowns were kept.

After some time, a technician led me to the huge radiation chamber filled with large machines. I was told to climb up on a slanted table, and lie on my stomach with my hands extended straight out above my head. This uncomfortable position created a backward arch that was hard to sustain for more than a few moments. If I were writing a prescription to cause lower back pain, this position would have fit the bill.

I was told not to move at all for what seemed like an eternity. The tech warned: "If you move we may harm you with the radiation or have to start all over again." The young technicians were quite limited in conversational skills and neither one explained what was about to happen. One technician asked the other: "Is this the correctly marked board for this patient? I don't see her name on it," comments that made me feel uneasy. The techs yanked the sheet under me, rolled me, and pushed my flesh to adjust my position. Occasionally I was asked to move my body up or sideways a ¼ centimeter on the board.

The techs spoke a foreign language of numbers and directions. One would say: "I got 89.5, I got 67. What do you have?" The other would answer: "I'm OK up and down," or "Let's shift her over a cm," while moving my buttocks or nudging my legs. They said they were marking me with permanent tattoos and taking port films. The absence of communication to me as a person felt dehumanizing. I know precision is important, but how about explaining things so the patient understands?

I have never felt more like a piece of meat on a slab in a butcher shop. A friend described her radiation experience as one of feeling violated. Blindsided by underestimating the difficulty of the experience because staff had not prepared me, I felt disoriented, frightened, and extremely uncomfortable. I felt ignored and upset that the techs didn't check how I was doing.

I finally blurted out: "Can you explain what you are doing now?" This led to only slightly more communication focused on the need for me to be still so I don't get mistreated. I felt my outstretched arms go numb and it was hard to get enough fresh air with my face in a downward position.

I heard a silent scream build inside of me and a desperate impulse to bolt off the table and say "I can't take this anymore." However, I restrained myself out of fear that they would have to start all over again. I tried to distract myself with regular breathing, humming tunes to drown out the annoying background music, and tapping my fingers. The techs wound up doing eight x-rays instead of the usual four. Am I so complicated, or did they make mistakes and unnecessarily x-ray me? I worried about the large volume of radiation to which I had already been exposed.

After nearly two hours of what was billed as a forty-minute session, I had to bend over the edge of the table to stretch in the opposite direction to reverse what had been done to my back. I felt spent and wiped out, already dreading future treatments. The experience was so horrible that I decided to report my experience to my doctor.

In subsequent weeks the radiation machines broke down several times per week, leading to rescheduling of patients. One morning I was called and told not to come that day, by noon I was told to come, and when I arrived at 3 pm, I was sent home again.

The breakdowns undermined my confidence in the machines and lent an amateurish feel to the operation. In addition, several inpatients were brought in for emergencies and "bumped" the waiting outpatients off schedule. As a result, wait times were close to two hours for a ten to fifteen minute appointment. Radiation had, in effect, become my daily afternoon activity.

Despite my frustration, I felt empathy for the technicians because they took their work seriously, often "power walking" between rooms to get things done quicker to meet their full schedule of patients every fifteen minutes. The work conditions surely pressured staff, making one wonder if accuracy was ever sacrificed for efficiency.

The patient waiting area had its own culture. The television blared noisily while some patients chatted with each other. I preferred reading, and wondered if anyone had considered a quiet waiting room for those patients who might want it. Conversations focused on patients' horror stories about their illness, bad treatment experiences, and daily life crises. Perhaps this was an unofficial support group, but I hadn't opted to join one. Besides, listening to venting about painful and traumatic experiences created negative energy, like second-hand smoke.

One day someone loudly told a story with gory details about a pit bull tearing into another dog and almost a child. When not assaulted by these stories one could overhear suggestive sounds of sicker patients vomiting right outside the waiting area. I wished I had brought ear plugs or blinders to block out the stimulus overload.

That particular afternoon I realized something felt very wrong for me. Being immersed in an atmosphere with such depressing auditory and visual stimuli made it hard to hold on to my cautious optimism about recovery and health. Moreover, for the pleasure of these daily ordeals I had to pay for parking. I reflected on the financial burden for poorer patients who couldn't afford it.

Despite my valiant efforts to stay afloat emotionally, I began to sink. Over time cumulative radiation irritated my bowels, creating significant digestive difficulties. I could hardly eat or drink without going to the bathroom immediately afterwards and each trip led to further irritation. I couldn't stand for a long time, nor could I sit down pain-free. A vicious cycle took over, leaving me a pretty miserable camper. I couldn't go out to walk, exercise, or worse yet, concentrate on writing, which was my lifeline. Some of these remnant physical side effects continued well past treatment.

My experience contradicted the 13th century Zohar's recommendation that the physician give the patient medicine for the body and the soul. Instead I felt battered by the treatment environment. As a last resort I recalled that: "The difference between try and triumph is a little "umph." I dug up whatever chutzpah I could muster and marched into the department manager and medical director's office to officially complain.

I hoped that my act of agency would help me and other patients as well. I was pleased when the new Manager of Operations of the Cancer Center welcomed my feedback. After our meeting, a water fountain, some candies, and additional reading materials appeared in the patient waiting area, gestures appreciated even by the staff.

I found that using my voice to speak up, complain, and identify deficiencies was an act of agency that strengthened me and even helped others. Becoming a "squeaky wheel," while not usually in my nature, was the necessary tool to obtain some constructive, albeit minor, improvements for patients.

February 7, 2007 – Done!

Things To Think About And Do

1. Trust your gut.

2. Journal your feelings, especially upsetting feelings.

3. Be patient with yourself but don't be too patient a patient!

4. Learn to ask questions and complain when necessary.

5. Do something fun or positive to counterbalance the negative stuff.

Chapter Eight

Surviving And Then What?

March 2007

After graduating from treatment I joined the growing ranks of cancer survivors who are cured or have their disease controlled.[1] I began to realize that survivorship is a new state of being that is never "done."[2] As others have discovered, life adjustment after cancer can present physical, psychological, social, and economic challenges.[3]

Surviving meant that cancer had left my body, but certainly not my mind. Cancer had taken away a sense of innocence and safety. Little physical symptoms that cropped up led a direct trail back to worry about possible recurrence. I was grateful for the frequent three month checkups that kept me closely monitored, and I didn't want the security of this umbilical cord cut.

The "new normal" included treatment side effects such as extreme fatigue, neuropathy and menopause. Others experience memory loss, different food tastes, cardiac issues, skin changes, and bone loss.[4] My slowly reappearing hair in unexpected shades of black and grey led me to cling to a wig for emotional security for over a year. Even after I looked more like myself I felt that friends and acquaintances related to me as if they saw a sign on my forehead saying "cancer patient," instead of viewing me as a person.

I was able to return to work part-time, then gradually full time. Fortunately, having my own private counseling practice meant that I didn't have to face negative experiences or reactions from co-workers in a larger workplace.[5] However, fatigue was a chronic companion that left me unable to get up early in the morning for work, like many other patients after treatment.

Patients returning to "normal" may experience a boat-load of emotions such as sadness, loss, and vulnerability, as well as spiritual angst. Mood swings, decrease in libido, anxiety over body image, and sensitivity to others' reactions are common.

One in four people with cancer have clinical depression, which may be an extension of their unending fatigue.

It was a steep adjustment going from three month checkups to longer intervals. Patients have described feeling left on their own, as busy doctors treating acutely ill patients have less time for long term survivors. When I saw sicker patients in the waiting room I felt a mixture of compassion, personal gratitude, and a tinge of survivor guilt as well.

I felt fortunate that my doctors continued to show concern for my physical and mental health. My wonderful oncologist reassured me that by doing aggressive treatment at the outset, the cancer was unlikely to recur. I credit my recovery to a combination of my doctors' quick response, my own efforts, and most importantly, to God's healing power.

I sometimes wondered how doctors deal emotionally with administering treatments that make patients suffer, and caring for patients who relapse and die. It takes a special spirit and commitment, but doctors are human too. One day after my three year checkup, I was shocked and disturbed to learn that my oncologist mysteriously resigned from his position and left town without warning. While the department offered alternative coverage, I felt sympathy for those patients who lost their doctor in the midst of treatment. It made me reflect on the toll the working environment can have on physicians who care for us.

When I shared my feelings about the oncologist's sudden departure with my gynecological surgeon, he replied in a tender, light-hearted way: "You don't need an oncologist any more. You don't need me either; we're just pretending." He was nudging me towards health, yet I was as thrown by his statement of wellness as by the loss of my oncologist.

My gynecologist always checked on how I was doing "in my head." He also inquired about any issues relating to sexual functioning after surgery and radiation, an often under-explored topic.[6] My homeopath recommended injections of mistletoe (Iscar), believed to suppress cancer cell growth and support T cell growth,[7] along with nutritional advice, and my acupuncturist supported me in regaining my energy.

Shedding my illness identity, unbecoming a "cancer patient," and returning to the land of the well was a confusing and gradual process. I wondered: is it like me being an alcoholic who is now "in recovery?" I felt stymied by a decision as small as where to park at the hospital lot before checkups. I would vacillate: do I park in the spaces reserved for cancer patients? At first I did, feeling my ordeal entitled me to the spot. Eventually I decided to leave spaces closer to the building for sicker patients, adding the benefit of a longer walk as I began to separate from my cancer identity.

Even after resuming normal life activities, returning to the land of the well included managing difficult memories and persistent anxieties. While family members are eager to move on and put the illness in the past, I had to nudge myself to embrace a personal mentality of health out of humility and caution, having watched several acquaintances who didn't survive. Like other cancer survivors, I had to grapple with the question of "how do I get my life back?" Shaping a meaningful future may include putting the illness in the past or learning to live alongside illness in the present.

Because "survivorship" is a significant stage, spiritual tools such as support groups and online forums can be excellent antidotes for unfinished emotional business and ongoing long-term needs. Discussion groups, relaxation techniques, yoga, physical therapy, meditation, acupuncture, biofeedback, and other modalities can be helpful. Patients can select an approach that meets their individual needs and temperament. Patients lacking adequate supports or with a history of maladaptive coping face greater vulnerability to psychological difficulties.

It is encouraging that many people experience a phenomenon of spiritual expansion and "post-traumatic growth" after treatment.[8] People who grow stronger and refuse to remain victims can be thought of as "triumphant survivors."[9] While I acknowledge emotional and spiritual growth, I am still working on a more confident attitude about the future. I have a need to give back to the world to express the deep gratitude I experienced.

I operationalized hope by making and looking forward to future plans. Sometimes rituals can help in this transition, such as saying the Hebrew *Shehecheyanu* prayer that expresses thankfulness to God for the privilege of reaching this moment. I also went to synagogue to say a *bircat gomel* prayer in front of the congregation. I hope and pray that I can stay in the land of the well for a long time as I continue to grow in strength and expand in spirit.

People are often curious to learn the end of the story: What happened to that patient struck with cancer? Did he survive? How is she doing? When I hear about acquaintances having serious illness it reminds me of my brush with frailty and mortality.

As I complete my story, I am now over seven years post treatment. "NED" (no evidence of disease) is the research marker defining cure. After cancer, one is exquisitely aware of the importance of the words of the Psalmist:

> *"Measure our days so we may acquire a heart of wisdom."*
>
> Psalm 90

Not only did time acquire new meaning for me, but focus on blessings and purpose in life was heightened.

My sojourning in the land of the sick has broadened my experience of life in so many ways. My understanding of suffering has expanded. My patience with the healing process has grown. My acceptance of my dependency on God and others has increased, as well as confidence in my own strength and self-reliance. Most of all, I live moment to moment. I appreciate the preciousness of life, feel grateful for my blessings, and seek inspiration to contribute to the world in my own unique way.

Things To Think About And Do

1. Remember that healing takes time.

2. Take it slow returning to work (if possible).

3. Reflect on how you are "doing" in your head.

4. Select a coping tool to help manage anxiety.

5. Identify supportive resources and seek them.

6. Explore a passion and begin it.

7. Express gratitude often.

8. Find new outlets and purpose.

9. Be hopeful and make future plans.

10. Be a "triumphant survivor."

Chapter Nine

Searching For Answers And Meaning

We can learn from everything in life, even from cancer cells. Those little troublesome cells were a red flag that shook me up to reflect on my life and nudged me in a new direction. I wouldn't go so far as to say "cancer was a blessing" but it certainly heightened my appreciation for the preciousness of life.

If you have experienced serious injury or illness you know that it is human nature to ask "why?" and even to seek something or someone to blame when one is dealt a short straw. I wasn't preoccupied with questions such as: "Is God angry with me?" "Is my suffering a punishment for some wrongdoing? "Why do good people suffer? "What is the meaning of life?", although many of these questions lurk in patients' minds, in search of answers.[1] Friends and family who can listen and be present can provide comfort even if they don't have answers.[2]

A search for answers may be unavoidable, but it can either be constructive or counter-productive. Engaging in a process of guilt, blame, and self-flagellation is of little value and can be harmful. By contrast, thoughtful self-examination can lead to positive restructuring of time and energy. It is up to each patient to accept the reality of what has happened and mobilize coping. I invite you to reflect on your situation to try to make some personal sense and meaning out of it.

Healthy coping includes creating meaning from an experience which lends some cognitive control over one's world.[3, 4] A frightening disease such as cancer with unclear etiology invites rampant speculation. One patient may believe in Divine intervention or fate, while another privileges genetics or environmental factors. Another may simply view illness as a case of "shit happens." Some patients identify factors outside themselves, while others look inwardly.

My intellectual curiosity to understand and make sense of situations prompted me to embark on a search for answers to see if I could learn something that could be meaningful for my future. Like an amateur detective I wanted to explore all angles – mind, body, and spirit, to understand what multi-determined factors beyond the random were at play. My questioning was personally helpful because it led to greater self-awareness. Tracking scientific research to learn about factors such as genetics, age, immunology, stress, lifestyle practices, and emotional functioning was eye opening for me.

From the field of genetic mapping we know that heredity plays a significant role in the transmission of illness tendencies. Dr. Samuel Hahnemann, the creator of homeopathic medicine, believed that each individual has a "Psora," a weakness or flaw in heredity that is like a genetic fault line under the surface.[5]

Hereditary tendencies such as the BRCA gene, can be discovered through genetic testing. Participation in studies using preventive screening tools to monitor hereditary family health conditions can help patients manage anxiety while demonstrating proactive agency for health.

From reading about genetic blood type differences and neurochemistry I learned that people like me, who have Type A blood, may have higher levels of cortisol (stress hormone). When we are healthy things remain benign, but under stress, inflammation can occur.[6] Blood types operate in conjunction with other factors, such as diet, stress, environmental conditions, and age. I had thought that my later menopausal age exerted a protective effect against bone loss and heart disease, only to learn that later age is a risk factor for uterine cancer; so much for aging gracefully.

I read that cancer grows faster under three circumstances:

1) A weakened immune system.
2) Chronic inflammation.
3) Development of blood vessels to feed tumor growth.

However, lifestyle choice interventions that counter these factors can transform the body's ability to resist cancer.[7] Ample research and popular opinion relate diet, exercise, nutrition, and environment to illness and health.[8] According to Servan-

Schreiber, genetic factors contribute at most 15% to our cancer risk; what we do or not do with our lives determines the other 85%. According to the World Health Organization, 80% of heart disease and 40% of cancers can be prevented with healthy diet and lifestyle.[9]

"The germ is nothing; the inner terrain is everything."
Louis Pasteur

Some have called cancer a four letter word – "ACID."[10] While these ideas may be controversial, they are gaining some momentum. The belief is that acidosis, caused by low pH foods, fatty tissue (an acid magnet), and stress are the main culprits in all disease. Fatty tissue stores acid to protect our organs, and tumors are actually "storage sheds" for acid. Wolfe believes that maintaining a balanced pH precedes the immune system as our first and major line of defense.

He advocates following an alkaline diet of simple, organic, complex carbohydrates, vegetables, especially from the mustard family, and avoiding refined flour, sugar, processed foods, animal fat, alcohol, soda, coffee, and beer, which create acidity. Not only our bodies, but also our environment seems to be growing progressively more acidic from toxic gases, emissions, and products we use in our homes.

The saying "you are what you eat" may actually be true. A ratio of 7 to 3 alkalinity/acidity is optimal for health.[11] As long ago as 1925, Nobel Prize winner Dr. Otto Warburg found that cancer cells thrive in (acidic) low oxygen states. By contrast, alkaline tissue holds twenty times more oxygen. A very alkaline body may be able to significantly raise the pH of malignant cells until they die. An oxygen-rich environment, therefore, is critical for maintaining health and reducing disease risk.

Richard Cabot, the founder of medical social work a century ago, wrote extensively about mind-body-social interaction.[12] Today, researchers link long-term stress with compromised immunity.[13] While stress doesn't cause disease, prolonged stress can worsen it. However, moderate levels of stress may actually have some positive benefit in activating our coping and bonding responses,[14] hence the value of programs that teach coping skills and offer group support to ease the patient's suffering.

Research concludes that "there is probably no organ system that is not influenced by the interaction between behavioral and physiological events,"[15] or in other words, our souls can affect our cells. Psycho-immunology research underscores the potential for held-in negative emotions to increase vulnerability, even toxicity in our system.[16, 17] These ideas were foreshadowed by the Baal Shem Tov, an 18th century Jewish mystic, who urged that in order to master our sorrows, we should immerse ourselves in and befriend emotions, but not be ruled by them.

Ed Friedman's integrative writing about psyche and soma suggests that psychological self-differentiation of the individual is related to immune system functioning.[18] Whatever stimulates differentiation of self can benefit the immune system, while factors such as dependency, avoiding challenge, and over-functioning suppress immune response.

Without an immune system, organisms lose integrity at a biological level. Friedman contends that emotional dynamics in systems can initiate and sustain pathology in a vulnerable member who is in a "malignant" position, such as being caught in noxious triangles between warring family members.

Friedman further distinguishes between Category I thinking (victimhood) and Category II thinking (responsibility), believing the latter fosters better coping because the individual's response of taking responsibility for his or her own health can potentially neutralize the hostility of an environmental stressor.[19]

Sacrificing caregivers are medically vulnerable because they are often unaware of their own stress levels while focusing so much on others. A woman caregiver for everyone in her multi-generational family came to see me when she became chronically ill. She quipped that: "the weak or meek shall inherit the earth because the strong die carrying them on their backs."[20] My mother was a strong healthy caregiver for my father, who was a cardiac patient for many years. She constantly worried about his health, eventually over-functioning for both of them. Perhaps not surprisingly, she died first and younger.

Stress and anxiety tend to narrow, even paralyze thoughtful

response, so tools that lower anxiety can foster clearer-headed thinking and flexible responses to help a person convert a crisis into an opportunity. Anxiety, the most prevalent contagious disease, keeps the body on constant alert and is the psychological correlate of inflammation on the physical level. Anxiety produces greater acidity in the body, and as we have learned, acidity and inflammation are linked to cancer cell development.

My homeopath, who has studied cancer research for decades, is concerned about acidity as well, but takes a broader view of cancer from a spiritual perspective as a disease of a person imprisoned in work or personal life, with the only freedom and spontaneity being expressed by cancer cells that follow no rules and wildly reproduce.[21] For this reason he encouraged me to reflect on my spiritual state and develop passionate goals as an antidote to drifting in life.

I reflected that the site of my cancer, the uterus, which is called *"rechem"* in Hebrew, comes from the word, *"rachamim,"* or compassion, I wondered: Was something going on with me compassion-wise? Did I have "compassion fatigue" for over thirty-five years of being present hour after hour for people's grief, despair, angst, fighting and bitterness? Was I too sensitive to their pain and taking too much responsibility for their healing? What about my over-functioning in my family and personal life as well? What kind of compassion was I showing myself by driving myself beyond my limits? Could all of this be taking a toll?

My pledge to transform my life became a guiding inspiration in recovery and afterwards. I needed to cope differently with anxiety in situations where I had no control. I could no longer feel so overly responsible for others, jumping in and trying to fix things. However, changing was not easy because I received praise and reinforcement for overdoing. Others complimented my over-functioning, such as in "you are so caring and capable," "How do you manage to do it all?" Yet I knew I needed to take the lead in doing something radically different.

I began employing a frequently used metaphor with clients of "taking one's temperature" with an imaginary thermometer to notice when stress felt too high and then making adjustments. I reflected that when a wild, undifferentiated process of cancer cell development is at large, the patient as a person, is not in charge. His or her body has been taken over, colonized, and weakened.

To counter these chaotic cells running the show, I needed to do something radically different. I began viewing the cells as immature, confused, and in need of the leadership I could provide through self-awareness, intuition, and self-expression. In their weakened state, they would be no match for a self-guided host.

Gratitude and refocusing on purpose became even stronger impulses guiding me. I was grateful that the primitive cancer cells, ordinarily found in the tiny ovaries, had instead been in the more self-enclosed uterus. I was grateful for the care from my doctors, support team, and friends. I was grateful for my husband and wonderful family, and especially the blessing of becoming a grandmother of twin girls.

My search for answers led me to conclude that many physical, emotional, and spiritual factors could be involved in illness, but that I would never know for certain as answers to many questions were unknowable. However, my search led me to create new meaning by focusing on God's purpose for us on earth: to be partners in the holy work of repairing our broken world, as each of us has a song, task, or mission to contribute.

This is where a Practical Spiritual approach comes in: equipping yourself with a set of spiritual coping tools that engage mind, body, and spirit can expand your perspective and vision, and help develop new meaning and purpose in life. We may never understand the meaning of our suffering, but each of us is invited to construct something positive out of our travails and go forward in life. Seeking a meaningful life and using our unique God-given talents to help repair the world was the answer to my search.

Things To Think About And Do

1. Keep your search for meaning constructive.

2. Reflect on your feelings and spiritual questions without judging yourself.

3. What meaning can you find about your illness from a spiritual point of view?

4. Learn information about your condition and research healthy lifestyle tips.

5. Manage your stress.

6. Don't over-function; learn to "take your temperature."

7. Make a future-oriented life plan.

8. Seek new purpose and find a passion.

9. Find a way to put your illness in perspective.

Chapter Ten

Healing Lessons And Practical Advice For Patients And Practitioners

My personal illness journey navigating the medical system, combined with patient care for many years as a mental health professional, taught me important healing lessons that can benefit patients and the practitioners who treat them. I feel personally blessed and grateful to have found doctors who listened to my needs, honored me as a person, and helped me feel like a partner in treatment. I hope that all doctors take time to answer patients' questions and ask patients how they are doing in their heads and hearts, not just in their bodies. Moreover, it is important that practitioners show a willingness to engage in spiritual conversations with patients.

What I learned about healing came to me on multiple tracks, like a sophisticated audio-visual system. I learned cognitively through reading and research, emotionally through personal experience, and spiritually through an open heart. My observations from working with groups of patients facing medical illness helped me understand that patients need an individualized approach to treatment.

I conducted an informal survey asking people what quality they most value in physician, clergy, therapist, or helpful friend. The most frequently-cited answer was "being there when I need them." A simple concept lacking technical jargon, "being there" is experienced as caring that is respectful, supportive, and empowering.[1] In times of loss, for example, the most appreciated help is often a friend who provides a steadying influence by just "being there."

> *"It rarely happens in life that you have a person who really understands what you are up against and openly faces it with you. That is what we can do for our patients and it is an enormous thing."*
>
> Michael Balint, pioneering English physician

I learned the importance of "being there" from a patient of mine who was desperately struggling with a mysterious and debilitating chronic illness. She told me that my "being there" created a special place and time that helped her feel validated and held emotionally. She used our sessions to share her painful burdens, feel understood, and learn about self-care.

Physicians who equate helping with tangible "doing" may be quick to dispense medicine, an approach certainly not lost on drug companies. If nothing concrete can be "done," a physician's lack of options can lead to the patient feeling a sense of abandonment. Time pressures in today's high tech medicine unfortunately work against spending quality time with patients to cultivate relationships. In situations of chronic and terminal illness, the ability to "be there" is especially important. In those situations adopting the reverse mantra may be helpful: "Don't just do something, sit there!"

"Being There"

At the heart of healing, like the hub of a wheel, is the practitioner's stance of "being there." Practitioners who can "be there" give patients the greatest gift; that's why it's called Presence. "Being there" means the ability to listen deeply, offer compassionate understanding, and provide guidance when needed. Encouraging the patient to speak not only about symptoms, but about life matters and concerns broadens the physician's understanding of the patient as a person. Being with a patient in an accepting manner is comforting and powerfully life affirming.

Beyond "Being There"

What are the elements of healing beyond "being there?" Healing is a slow process that moves from the inside out. Time is required to step back and reflect on one's path and how to change it. Healing means different things to different people, and can be accessed through a variety of pathways. Healing involves new viewing and doing, and healing involves taking charge of one's destiny. Having a large repertoire of down-to-earth spiritual tools creates a wider perspective with options that can lead to more flexible coping. Healing and becoming healthy is more than just the absence of disease and recovering from illness. Health is a state of mind; being healthy involves handling stress in positive ways and reacting creatively to inevitable change.

Seven Tips And Healing Practices
For Patients To Adopt

Lesson I – Take personal responsibility

> *"It is what it is. We can't change it; we have to decide how we are going to respond. We cannot change the cards we are dealt; just how to play the hand."*
>
> Randy Pauch's last lecture[2]

Whatever caused the illness (e.g. genetics, lifestyle habits, bad luck...) it is up to you to develop a coping response. What matters is how we respond to stress and what tools and resources we employ in our own self-defense. A helpless victim mentality won't stimulate resilience. Resilience involves focusing on beliefs and actions to help us break out of a negative cycle, and finding positive meaning in negative situations. Take personal ownership of your responses to stress and be your own agent.

Lesson II – Listen and learn from your heart

> *"Your heart will give you greater counsel than all the world's scholars."*
>
> Talmud

If we approach the illness crisis as presenting both danger and opportunity, we can view it as a potential growth experience from which we can learn about ourselves and life. A change of heart is required: Cultivate gratitude as if it were a garden! I am grateful for what I learned about myself, and for the new growth and life attitudes that emerged from my illness experience. Listen to the intuitive wisdom of your inner spirit and the emotional wisdom of your heart. Pursue new dreams in an open-hearted way and make plans for a healthy life now.

Lesson III – Express yourself with new authentic self-talk

We need to revise negative views of ourselves and our lives by affirming the good and sacred in each of us. We need to change the stories we tell ourselves. The language and self-talk we use are crucial, especially when putting stress in perspective. For example when dealing with frustrations, one can say: "I'm having root canal surgery, but it's not cancer," or "I had a social disappointment, but it's not cancer."

New self-talk can create a more mature perspective. Stop complaining about minor things, and don't sweat the small stuff. Use positive self-instructions for encouragement, such as the ones I gave myself: "Slow down and rest; think good thoughts; be patient with yourself; picture yourself well; and remember, others care and think about you." Express positive affirmations to yourself and remind yourself that you matter.

You are a child of God.

Your playing small doesn't save the world.
There's nothing enlightened about
shrinking so that other people
won't feel insecure around you. We are
all meant to shine, as children do.
We were born to make manifest
the glory of God that is within us.
It's not just in some of us; it's in Everyone.

And, as we let our own light shine,
we unconsciously give other people
permission to do the same.
As we are liberated from our fear,
our presence automatically
liberates others.

© Marianne Williamson [3]

Lesson IV – Learn to Be Flexible

You can re-write your own life script. The straits of illness are narrow; seek wider paths through revising attitudes and behavior. Opening yourself to new options, alternatives, and pathways that can lead to greater flexibility and foster healing. For example, I cannot stress enough that learning to accept help is as important as giving it. Things that had to be "just so" or "perfect" can really be "another way" or even "good enough." You aren't a machine, but rather an evolving human organism that can adapt, expand, and change. Those who don't adapt, won't survive. Learn flexibility, seek alternatives, and learn to go with the flow.

Lesson V- What you do does make a difference

The illness crisis and detour can be an opportunity to take the road less traveled. Doing things the old way means no change; trying new behaviors can lead to different experiences and outcomes. Setting short and long-term goals with concrete action steps embodies hope. Even if you start doing something without initial conviction, the doing of it can lead to new meaningful outcomes. Focus energy on reaching your goals to build self-confidence. Use coping tools to manage fear, reduce helplessness, and increase agency, connection, and well-being. Carving out time to care for yourself affirms your value. Start now to create new experiences and outcomes; Just do it.

Lesson VI – Don't Go it alone

> *"If you want to go fast, go alone. If you want to go far, go together."*
>
> African proverb

"Lone Rangers" are not to be emulated; even the Lone Ranger had his friend Tonto for help and support. Illness reminds us that we cannot be islands; we need others to help us heal. Remember that it takes a village. Embrace caring friends and community who reach out to help you. When I was going through treatment, having a supportive team helped me feel less alone and more cared about.

Each part of the "village" had a different task: A listening ear, a humor coach, a good medical question asker, a meal organizer, and a social connector. Together they composed a beautiful fabric of support that strengthened me. If you are ever in doubt about leaning on others, remember that helping makes the helper feel good too. Don't isolate yourself like an island when you need a village of helpers to act as a team on your side.

Lesson VII - Accept what the universe presents

The universe is filled with blessing and suffering. We must accept that reality as a first step, because we can't cope well with something if we deny or fight its reality. For example, when Nancy Reagan was informed of her malignancy, her comment was: "I guess it's my turn; that's the human condition."

A beautiful poem written by Rachel Tova Minkove expresses the vulnerability and fragility of life that she knew only too well in her long courageous struggle with illness.

Roller Coaster

Up and down, up and down
The roller coaster glides through time,
Each day feeling like an eternity.
The passenger shrieks as the coaster reaches its highest elevation,
Knowing full well what comes next.
The dreaded drop.

At the lowest point, the passenger emits a whitish hue
And is ready to get off this frightening journey.
The only thing holding her back is the exhilaration of staying high forever.
Is that a possibility?
She ponders.
The passenger has quickly learned that
***Anything** is possible in this roller coaster of life.*
Rachel Tova Minkove, 2008, (d.2012)

In truth, we humans don't control the strings of the world and it is helpful to develop a humble attitude. Any of us is just one tick away from having our lives change in ways that we could never imagine. Our challenge, therefore, is to make every day count. Cherish your family and friends, enjoy them while you have them, and relish life while you have it; that is the secret recipe for joy. Accept the mixed blessings the universe presents with grace and humility and learn to "let it go and let God in," or in the words of the inimitable Beatles' song: "Let it be."

I hope these healing lessons and the following quote will offer you inspiration on your journey.

> *I am the hero of my own life story – I will behave like one.*
> *I won't dwell upon the past; the past is over.*
> *I will be the one, the only one, in charge of my future.*
> *I will be patient – nothing happens all at once – but not passive.*
> *I will trust in a Higher Power to help me along the way.*
> *And – I will trust in myself.*

Rabbi Maurice Lamm
The Power of Hope [4]

Things To Do Think About And Do

1. Explain your needs to those who treat you.

2. Expect to be able to ask questions and collaborate with your doctor.

3. Trust in yourself because your future is your responsibility.

4. Listen to your heart and focus on gratitude.

5. Learn to express yourself in positive ways.

6. Give up perfectionism, and know that God doesn't make junk either.

7. Try to be flexible and embrace doing new things.

8. Assemble a village of support.

9. Accept what life presents.

10. Be the hero/heroine of your life story.

PART III
A DOWN-TO-EARTH
SPIRITUAL TOOLBOX

Chapter Eleven

An Alphabet Of Practical Spiritual Coping Tools

I hope it has been helpful following my diary and learning how I used a variety of spiritual tools to cope and renew my spirit during illness, treatment, and recovery. In the next section I will describe an alphabetical treasure chest of spiritual tools available for your use. The tools are from complementary and alternative medicine, creative expression, inspirational wisdom, meditative practices, nature, prayer, Psalms, rituals, stories, texts, and *tikkun olam.*

I know I am not alone in turning to spiritual tools during difficult times. Over the centuries people have used these tools to cope and heal from illness, trauma, and personal crisis. Having a repertoire of inner and outer resources helps people face challenges with greater flexibility and self-confidence. These tools integrate an ethereal spiritual dimension with down-to-earth behavioral practices that tap into emotional experience, provide comfort and inspiration, and lift one's spirits. My perspective is that they are not just spiritual tools, but through their active use, provide psychological benefits that enhance coping. I hope you will reflect on which ones appeal to you. Any or all of them can make a difference, not just during illness, but in cultivating a healthy lifestyle.

Complementary And Alternative Approaches

Increasing numbers of patients turn to Complementary and Alternative Medicine (CAM) with its holistic approach to mind, body, and spirit. This integrative form of medicine helps people feel empowered and involved in their own care by encouraging patients to take active, responsible steps toward healthy practices.[1] I believe that the focus on prevention, meaningful doctor-patient relationships, and a spiritual dimension are social factors that contribute to healing.

Research documents the benefits of complementary and

alternative medicine in handling side effects of medical treatment, reducing distress, boosting immunity, and improving quality of life. For example, acupuncture helped me feel more balanced and supported during and after chemotherapy. Meditation and guided imagery help many people adjust their reactivity and arousal levels to achieve greater emotional self-regulation.

Because of these experienced benefits, it should not be surprising that Americans spend huge sums of money on CAM,[2] and a growing number of leading hospitals now offer a range of unconventional therapies once spurned by mainstream medicine.[3] The growing demand for these treatments from a majority of cancer patients has forced their greater acceptance by the traditional medical establishment.

The American Cancer Society has provided a *Complete Guide to Complementary and Alternative Cancer Therapies.* Unfortunately, patients often pursue complementary treatments without telling their doctors for fear of disapproval. I wish biomedical and alternative practitioners could communicate to avoid contradictory interventions with unintended consequences.

For example, while many recommended alternative treatments are safe, certain practices might interfere with chemotherapy.[4] Herbs, for example, can intensify the impact of medicines, causing adverse reactions.[5] For that reason, I believe that an integrated collaborative approach between disciplines would benefit the patient.

Acupuncture

Acupuncture, one of the most widely researched and accepted complementary approaches, stimulates specific points on meridians (energy channels of the body) using thin sterile needles manipulated by hand or electrical stimulation with the aim of improving and balancing levels of Qi ("chee"), the vital energy of life. Acupuncture releases hormone-like chemicals that can affect one's mood, perception of pain, and brain mechanisms involved in inflammation and immune functioning.

Acupuncture helps patients suffering from back pain, osteo-arthritis, post-operative pain, and some of the side effects of chemotherapy, such as nausea.[6] In addition, the healing aspects of acupuncture include the relationship with the practitioner, expectation of benefit, and the emotional support provided.[7] Visits to my acupuncturist provided a welcomed outlet for me to express and release emotions and worries.

Homeopathy

Developed by Samuel Hahnemann in the 1700s, homeopathy focuses on the body's own healing responses, employing a vaccine-like principle of "like cures like" and using remedies that come from plants, minerals, and animals.

I routinely consult with a homeopath as a "check and balance" to standard biomedical interventions. He typically supports and complements my biomedical efforts, at times offering homeopathic and lifestyle interventions. For example, given my aggressive cancer, he endorsed the "big guns" of chemo (a systemic process) over local radiation, and encouraged me to return for homeopathic support (with Iscar) once my treatments were over.

His four-pronged approach to cancer consists of: 1) dealing with the tumor; 2) cleansing the body of toxins; 3) prescribing nutritional improvements; 4) changing habits of mind and heart that reflect being "stuck" in life. He emphasizes the importance of an alkaline diet, eating whole foods, and staying away from products that increase acid in the body such as red meat and sugar, because it is true that "you are what you eat!"

Ayurveda

Ayurveda is a 5,000-year-old system of natural medicine long practiced in India. Ayurveda teaches balance in lifestyle, and views optimal digestion as the key to good health and long life. For example, when we don't digest our food or have enough good bacteria, the condition resulting is imbalance and weak digestive fire, often manifested in symptoms of gas and bloating. Ayurveda uses interventions with herbs and other modalities to remedy unhealthy conditions.

Massage And Touch

*"The way to health is a scented bath and an oiled massage
every day."*

Hippocrates, 4th century

Massage, with roots in antiquity 3,000 years ago, is an extremely popular practice throughout the world and a significant form of health care in many countries. In the United States today, 85,000 practitioners give sixty million massage treatments each year to twenty-five million Americans.[8] Massage is used for comfort, stress reduction, pain management, rehabilitation, movement training, and palliative care.

Massage is not only tactile, but also involves the powerful sense of smell. People are drawn to massage because it benefits circulation, muscle relaxation, and hormonal and immune systems. Rats undergoing belly massage release oxytocin, and AIDS patients' natural killer cells increase after several massages. Skilled practitioners use their hands to sense a patient's energy fields as they administer therapeutic touch. Reflexology is another related approach in which trained practitioners manipulate areas on the bottom of the feet to clear energy blockages and produce well-being.

Judiciously used therapeutic touch is valuable and can be comforting to patients because it communicates an important message: "You are cared about and touchable," a message that contradicts what cancer patients often feel, that is, being untouchable. While in the hospital after my abdominal surgery I held a silk pillow against my stomach for support when I took my first painful steps of recovery. I also used it as a foot and head rest, and hugged it for comfort. Inscribed with a picture of Jerusalem and the words, *"El na refa na la"* (Please God, heal her, please) and a *"hamsa,"* (a Middle Eastern symbol for long life and prosperity), it lifted my spirits as well.

We gave a similar pillow to one of the gravely ill patients in our support groups. He held for comfort during his last days in the hospital. After his death, his young daughter found comfort by holding her father's pillow when she missed him. Realizing how special this pillow could be, I began calligraphing decorated pillows with the words, "Please God Heal Her/Him, Please" in Hebrew or English. I enclose prayers, Psalm verses, or messages tailored to the person's religion and relevant to the person's situation. When I give the pillow to friends or strangers undergoing illness, surgery, or chemo, the pillow acts as a long-distance hug that provides spiritual inspiration. Other projects, such as giving patients blankets, shawls, and comforters, communicate to them that "we are knitted together" and "blanketed by Divine love."[9] Patients are deeply touched by these gifts, and appreciate the comfort and caring.

Yoga

Yoga, an ancient meditative practice that predates formal religion, is a physically active spiritually-based activity involving stretching, postures, and movement. Yoga styles and techniques vary, from gentle yoga to more intense "hot" Bikram yoga. Used to "yoke" the mind, yoga activates the parasympathetic nervous system to reduce adrenaline-fueled reactions to stress. Nerves send signals throughout the body to slow the heart rate, and brain imaging studies show positive elements when people hold yoga poses.[10] I found gentle and restorative yoga to be a wonderful mind-body practice that helps my posture, flexibility, mind, and spirit all at once.

Creative Expression

Art

"Art washes away from the soul the dust of everyday life."
Pablo Picasso

I value creative expression because it engages both sides of the brain and stimulates insight and healing. Art can dramatize one's dilemmas by communicating inner experience. For example, a picture I drew of myself carrying two heavy suitcases helped me realize that I was shouldering too much worry for others and needed to do more self-care. For me, art is an intensely engrossing and spiritually gratifying adventure with an almost meditative quality. While engaged in art, hours can pass without my awareness of time.

My colleague and I used a form of artistic expression called Handmade Midrash[11] in our spiritual/study discussion groups. It involved cutting or tearing pieces of colored paper and gluing them to make a two or three dimensional collage based on a biblical text. After reading the 23rd Psalm together, each participant assembled a collage based on a verse he or she found meaningful. One person used the verse "You prepare a table for me in the presence of my enemies" and designed a table under which he hid in fear of his wife's imminent death. He sought shelter "in the house of the Lord." Another participant assembled a "cup runneth over" to signify her need to learn to set limits. A third created a pastoral scene with palm trees "by still waters" to calm her spirits. With the same Psalm participants expressed themselves uniquely through art.

Mosaic art can be a metaphor for the illness experience. The broken pieces of glass, plastic or even paper represent the trauma that shattered safety and created "brokenness." The pieces can then be assembled to form a beautiful new design, symbolically mirroring the healing process. In the Bible, Moses was commanded to carry the broken tablets of the Ten Commandments in the Holy Ark together with the new ones to show that God cares about a shattered world and accepts people broken by sickness, disability, pain, trauma, or loss. Since none of us is without some form of brokenness that needs healing, we must gently carry those broken parts of ourselves and embrace all members of the community, whatever their condition in life.

Humor, Play, Laughter

"What soap is to the body, laughter is to the soul."

Yiddish saying

Serious illness depresses us and creates difficult vulnerable emotions which can further suppress our immune systems. Humor and laughter can lighten our spirits and help us not take ourselves too seriously. Activities that stimulate fun can decrease negative feelings, improve coping, and help us feel more alive.[12] Laughter is a stress buster, mood lifter, and people connector.[13] Norman Cousins called laughter the best medicine, claiming that ten minutes of daily belly laughing had an anesthetic effect and helped him sleep.[14] Laughter releases endorphins, increases circulation and right brain thinking, relaxes muscles and blood vessel walls, and lowers risk of heart disease.

> *"Laughter is the shortest distance between people."*
>
> Victor Borge

> *"A cheerful heart makes for good health."*
>
> Proverbs 17:22

> *"Even in the pit of hell, it is a mitzvah to be joyful."*
>
> Reb Nachman of Breslov

The prophet Isaiah consoled his exiled people by urging them to:

> *"Rejoice with joy and singing."*
>
> Isaiah 35:2

Martha Washington, who lived through the American Revolution, was twice widowed, and buried four of her children, understood that the greater part of happiness or misery depends more on our disposition than our circumstances.

Ken Blanchard points out the connection between "ha-ha" and "a-ha," suggesting that humor can lead to insight. In addition to humor, a sense of feistiness can be useful. While feisty or complaining patients are often unpopular with medical staff, these "squeaky wheels" are better at getting attention than are mild mannered, cooperative patients.

Katherine Hepburn once quipped:

> *"If you obey all the rules, you miss all the fun."*

> *"When humor goes, there goes civilization."*
>
> Irma Bombeck

Journaling

"Writing gives us agency: we are not acted upon by a situation; we are acting. We are no longer being 'done to' by the illness; we are doing." [15]

Peggy Penn

Journaling was an important creative outlet that helped me record my thoughts and feelings. The actual writing slowed down emotional process and fostered greater self-awareness. Journaling made me aware of disabling emotional and behavioral habits that needed changing, such as over-functioning. Writing down feelings can be a first step in promoting new actions. For example, getting in touch with angry feelings can lead to saying "no" and setting appropriate limits where needed.

Research has found that journaling gives a person a voice. Cathartic expression through writing, especially about upsetting experiences, actually increases T-cell counts and immune function. [16] While you can handwrite, type, or record orally, I personally find writing by hand more direct in downloading and validating my feelings. To begin journaling, try reflecting on an event and take note of the feelings it evoked, or write a feeling word (such as "sad," "afraid") and free associate to the word. You may also find that writing with the non-dominant hand brings out more vulnerable emotions.

Music

"To groan when ill is common; to sing when ill is courageous."

HaRav Kook

There is an almost universal responsiveness to music. Hearing is one of the last senses retained by brain-damaged and dying patients, even when they can no longer speak or process language. [17] Whether instrumental or vocal, music puts us in touch with our deeper selves and our own natural rhythmic instrument – the body. [18] Even moaning can be self-soothing to a worn out patient.

Music has a long tradition in the healing arts. Certain sounds decrease stress symptoms of rapid heart rate, shallow breathing, and adrenalin release.[19] Wordless melodies (*"niggunim"*) can produce a relaxed meditative state.[20] This may explain why harp music is often used to create a soothing atmosphere for dying patients. In contemporary medicine, Gaynor uses sounds of Tibetan singing bowls to foster "entrainment" (attunement or harmony) for cancer patients.[21] We used music and singing as important elements to set a reflective mood and foster connection in our spiritual study/discussion groups.

> *"In order to strengthen the vital powers, one should employ musical instruments and tell patients gay stories which will make their hearts swell."*
>
> Maimonides

I enjoy musical expression and participate in a Klezmer musical group called The Tummelers ("those who make a joyful noise"). When we perform at senior centers and we distribute toy instruments to the elderly and disabled patients, I find it heartwarming to watch them shake the instruments as they recognize old tunes from their youth in Eastern Europe. While these encounters sadly remind me of the impact of aging, they also demonstrate the power of music to engage and elevate the spirit.

> *"It is good to make a habit of inspiring yourself with a melody ... for the loftiness of melody is beyond all measure."*
>
> Reb Nachman of Breslov

The Jewish sages long ago knew the power of music and song to mobilize and lift the spirit. Contemporary spiritually-based music resonates with people facing hard times. For example, when my colleague and I made brief pastoral visits to hospitalized patients, we often played soothing music such as "Bridge Over Troubled Water." Patients easily related the song to their illness and life situation. They often voluntarily shared who or what was their "bridge" and what they needed for healing.

Humming music while I walk helps me pay attention to my inner mood and helps me feel less alone. When I pushed my little granddaughters in a tree swing, I found myself singing the simple, but profound tune "Row, row, row your boat." The song mirrored the gentle rocking, my joy in being with them in those precious moments of mutual adoration.

Poetry

Poetry is a true language of the heart that conveys emotion in a concentrated way. My father was a quiet, reserved physician with a spiritual, but anti-religious bent. When my mother became terminally ill, he burst forth with powerful poetry as a way of coping with overwhelmed feelings. After my mother's death, he wrote seven books of poetry that served as a therapeutic outlet for healing life-long traumas.

At the Window of the Hospital

A small figure with pipes
going into and out of her body,
a shadow of a sad smile on her face.

The window in front of which
I silently stood
has become to me a Holy Ark,
and my lips murmured a prayer.

A flock of birds landed in the park,
They stood in rows and said
a "Prayer for the Road."

Suddenly, they departed
and flew into blue distance.

She smiled
And I knew

That the prayers
were favorably received.

George Gorin © 1980

Security

I am her support
and rock of security,
and she clings to me...

And we both hover
over the edge
of a precipice.

George Gorin
George Gorin © 1980

Inspirational Wisdom

"It is gratefulness which makes the soul great."
Rabbi Abraham Joshua Heschel

Words we say reflect our values and shape our moods. I collect quotes and sayings that resonate with me and put them on my desk wall where I can be reminded of them. Sometimes I carry a saying in my wallet. Selecting even one word or mantra such as "believe" or "hope" can inspire our thoughts and energies constructively. Actively reciting positive affirmations can lift mood and cultivate gratitude for blessings, an emotional attitude that can transform us and make us better and often happier people.

One of the first quotes I collected when I took ill was a reminder to honor one's body, a responsibility long emphasized in Jewish tradition. We get one body in this life. Despite today's technological advances that can replace many body parts, much like a car being fixed in an auto repair shop, how we care for our bodies will impact how long and well they last.

> *"The body is a sacred garment. It's your first and last garment: it is what you enter life in and what you depart life with; it should be treated with honor."*
>
> Martha Graham

The essence of a spiritual attitude is the ability to pay attention and appreciate the present moment. While it is certainly human to anticipate the future and regret past disappointments, I admire the ability to live life by going with the flow.

To paraphrase a clever saying credited to Eleanor Roosevelt:

> *"Yesterday is history; tomorrow is a mystery, but today is a gift; that's why it's called the Present."*

Interestingly, the word "serenity" is found within the word "serendipity." Serendipity is a way of living as if everything is a miracle and potentially positive. While I am a planner, I try to seize the moment and be open to when opportunities present themselves, embracing the idea that "coincidences are God's way of remaining anonymous."

> *"You cannot discover new oceans unless you have the courage to lose sight of the shore."*
>
> Andre Gide

Healing and growth come from within and often involve a difficult process of taking new risks. Making changes can be fraught with ambivalent emotions. Several quotes gave me sustained inspiration during my spiritual recovery.

> *"Everything great begins with a dream. Whatever you can do, or dream you can, begin it. Boldness has genius, power, and magic in it."*
>
> Goethe

"The future belongs to those who believe in the beauty of their dreams."

Eleanor Roosevelt

"Never doubt that a small group of thoughtful, committed citizens can change the world. Indeed it is the only thing that ever has."

Margaret Mead

When facing difficult times such as illness, finding courage to face one's fears may be the key ingredient. Eleanor Roosevelt once said:

"You gain strength, courage, and confidence by every experience in which you really stop to look fear in the face. You are able to say to yourself, 'I have lived through this horror. I can take the next thing that comes along.' You must do the thing you think you cannot do."

Dave Barry adds a lighthearted prodding to find courage to do new things when he wrote:

"Never be afraid to try something new. Remember, amateurs built the ark; professionals built the Titanic."

Gordon Livingstone, a man who suffered numerous losses, reminds us:

"We are never without choices, no matter how desperate the circumstance ... all is not lost. We are not dead yet."

Sick patients may tend to withdraw from socializing, even though connections can be an important source of support and strengthening.

Proverbs urge:

"When a person has a heavy heart let him speak it out to others."

A Japanese proverb also reminds us of the strength and value of community:

"A single arrow is easily broken, but not ten in a bundle."

The inspiring Helen Keller said:

"Alone we can do so little; together we can do much."

The great first century sage Hillel stated:

"If I am not for myself, who will be for me? If I am only for myself, what am I? And if not now, when?"

This statement encourages us to think of self-care, helping others, and adopting these important practices NOW.

Meditative Practices; Mindfulness, Visualization, Guided Imagery

"Much silence makes a mighty noise."

African proverb

Meditation is a 5,000-year-old Eastern practice that has established a major foothold today in Western culture with millions of meditators in North America.[22] Meditation is an umbrella term for diverse self-regulatory practices emphasizing focused attention on the breath, thereby leading to greater self-awareness and emotional balance. Meditation often uses some mantra (sound, word, or phrase recited repetitively, or in unvarying tone) as an object of concentration. Because no two meditative practices are alike, meditation is difficult to standardize and research.

Herb Benson's early research on Transcendental Meditation found that it counteracted stress by decreasing blood pressure, breathing rate, and metabolism, leading to lowered anxiety and reactivity.[23] Meditation reduces internal judgmental chatter,[24] clears the mind, and enables greater self-observation. Meditation can help us be gentler with ourselves and set more realistic expectations. Relaxation can foster deeper listening and confidence in self-management.[25] Other benefits include creating a sense of refreshment, relaxation, and changed perspectives on problems.

It is known that meditation increases brain activity and can improve physiological functioning and create wellbeing.[26] Thanks to our brain's circuitry, meditation, intense contemplation, repetitive prayer or ritual can actually stimulate the brain to experience a sense of union and spiritual connection outside the self.[27] In fact, scientists have found structural differences in the brains of meditators, the latter showing slow, focused waves similar to those found during sleep.[28]

The Dalai Lama XIV believed that there was no need for temples or complicated philosophy. Instead, he considered our brains and hearts to be our temple, using a philosophy of kindness.[29]

The Buddha, ("one who is aware") taught a variety of spiritual practices to awaken the mind and open the heart, develop loving-kindness, generosity, and moral integrity. His method involved focusing on the breath and body to become aware of one's feelings and moods. He urged mastering one's senses and quieting the body and mind in order to be free.

> *"Meditation before God brings forth the holy spark that is found in every individual."*
>
> Reb Nachman of Breslov

From a Jewish spiritual perspective, our breath connects us to the rhythms of the universe. God's transfer of breath into Adam implies that all life is sacred and depends on God. Breathing, therefore, can connect a person with his or her Divine inner spark.

According to Rabbi Kerry Olitzky, during addiction, an addict's Divine spark is hiding beneath the surface, growing nearly cold, but still there.

Turning to God in meditation as part of the recovery process can fan the Divine spark back into flames and subdue the addictive drive.[30]

> *"You are wherever your thoughts are. Make sure your thoughts are where you want to be."*
>
> Reb Nachman of Breslov

Visualization and Guided Imagery

Visualization is a meditative practice that harnesses the extraordinary power of the mind. Adding sensory imagery generated by the individual creates an altered state in which beliefs and attitudes can change. Each person has self-healing abilities and the conscious/unconscious knowing of what is needed for healing. Visualizations can generate powerful emotional experience, and scientists tell us that using our minds to imagine doing an activity can activate the same neural circuits as actually doing that activity.

Guided imagery can help a person access a calm state, find strength and greater self-acceptance. For example, one patient who was anxious about beginning chemotherapy visualized herself as Dr. Superwoman before each treatment to help her face her fears more courageously. An extensive library of books and CD's offer visualizations to help patients with a range of health conditions, medical treatments, and maintaining wellness.

In creating imagery relating to cancer it is helpful to portray treatment as a strong ally and powerful friend who repairs damage, and to portray cancer cells as weak and confused. Achterberg cautions against creating too intense images of cancer cells.[31] Instead, she suggests visualizing white blood cells as the patient's team or army functioning as a Quality Control System to weed out cancer cells. I visualized cancer cells melting away, shrinking, or evaporating, rather than being devoured by PacMan, a popular earlier metaphor.

A colleague diagnosed with breast cancer developed her own healing visualization. Before her double mastectomy she went to the seashore to immerse herself in the ocean. She imagined being in a *mikveh*, and visualized her body being cleansed and healed physically, emotionally, and spiritually as the water surrounded her and carried away the illness and anything else she wanted to get rid of.

Beautiful images of shelter in liturgy can be used as visualizations to help people manage fears and feel less alone. For example, the metaphor of *"Sukkat Shelomecha"* conjures up being sheltered under the roof of the *sukkah*, signifying God's protection of the Israelites as they wandered in the desert. Another enveloping image is "under the wings of the *Shekhinah.*"

When people are ill, the image of childhood maternal care can be very comforting. A powerful nurturing image is found in: "Blessed Be God, who *holds* me to Her Breast when I am broken and cradles me when my body and spirit ache."[32] A patient of mine created an image of being held and rocked in a "God sack" to soothe her fears. Other religious traditions have comforting images as well, such as being surrounded by the folds of Mary's mantle.

Visualizations can be particularly helpful to a person at night when lying still, a time when awareness of bodily processes, symptoms, and discomfort can let imagination run wild and heighten anxiety. One beautiful musical visualization crafted by the late cantor and song writer Debbie Friedman,[33] portrays the four angels within Jewish tradition surrounding and protecting the patient with their benevolent qualities: *Michael*, (on the right) represents the likeness and compassion of God; *Gavriel*, (on the left) represents strength; *Uriel*, (in front) represents the light of God, and *Rephael*, (in back), the healing of God.

Hovering above is the presence of *Shekhinah*, creating a surround-sound effect with the patient being lovingly embraced and watched over by Divine protection. One can add hand motions to the words and melody, pointing in the direction of the specific angels while doing the visualization.

Nature

"I go to nature to be soothed and have my senses put in order."

John Burroughs

Human beings' relationship to nature has been a theme of poets and philosophers over the centuries. Contemplating the variety of colors, sounds, and shapes in nature can inspire a spiritual sense of awe that nurtures our souls and comforts us during difficult circumstances. Thinking about a pungent green forest, the broad silent whiteness of snow, a fresh gurgling brook, or a beautiful sunset, and stepping outside to touch nature, brings us closer to the wider universe of living things. From nature we can learn beauty, patience, and humility about our place in the universe.

"Ecological awareness is spiritual in its deepest sense – connecting all life to itself and to that which is greater."
Fritjof Capra

"Nature is so full of genius, full of divinity, that not a snowflake escapes its fashioning hand."
Henry David Thoreau

My father loved to tend his rose garden in the summer as it was the only time he escaped from the concrete jungle of work in the big city. He would nurture his climbing roses until they became a canopy of fragrant deep pink surrounding our deck. He wrote this poem about how nature can inspire a spiritual feeling of awe.

Transcendence

On a plateau surrounded by hills
you have a feeling of transcendence
and of nearness to Heaven and God

The beauty of background
suggests that the Creator
passed this place and adorned it
with a string of wooded hillocks
to give man tranquility of peace
and peace of security.

George Gorin
Echoes and Shadows © (1985), p10

Since I also find gardening to be a soul-feeding activity, I nourish my flowers with water and words of encouragement. My plants never talk back to me, but rather show their appreciation by growing well. When my garden is overgrown with weeds, I do "furious weeding" to vent frustrated emotions harmlessly.

"The art of healing comes from nature."

Paracelsus

Sue Patton Thoele suggests we imagine ourselves as flowers thirsty for care and appreciation, and grateful for sustaining feeding.[34] Because a compassionate inner environment allows us to bloom more beautifully, she encourages us to tend our inner garden by gently pruning limiting beliefs and actions.

When we face overwhelming circumstances, nature can be a comforting escape, while reminding us of the beauty of the world. When Anne Frank and her family hid in a secret annex in Amsterdam for two years during the German occupation of Holland in World War II, she would go up to the attic and gaze at the sky. Doing that helped her compensate for not being able to go outdoors lest she be discovered and deported to death. She wrote in her diary:

"The best remedy for those who are afraid, lonely, or unhappy, is to go outside, somewhere where they can be quite alone with the heavens, nature, and God. Because only then does one feel that all is as it should be and that God wishes to see people happy, amidst the simple beauty of nature. As long as this exists, and it certainly always will, I know that then there will always be comfort for every sorrow, whatever the circumstances may be."

Anne Frank[35]

In Jewish tradition there is a little known ancient sacred text called *Perek Shira*,[36] or Song of the Universe, attributed by some sources to King David, and by others to King Solomon, who was reputed to understand the "speech" of animals, vegetables, and minerals. Each component of creation (heavenly bodies, mountains, oceans, animals, birds, fish, and insects) has its own "song" as a way of praising God and impacting the world. While the word *"shira"* means song, its true meaning is task or function. The message is that every action matters, and people must also rise to their level of song to complete their mission on earth in fulfillment of God's will.

A Drop of Water

Even a drop of water
has a purpose
and a goal.

It breaks through rock
to reach a river
in order to become
a drop in the sea.

George Gorin
Intermezzo © (1984), p42

Reb Nachman of Breslov recommended nature as a place conducive to quieting the self and opening the heart.

God:
Grant me the ability to be alone!

May it be my custom to go outdoors each day
among the trees and grass
among all growing things,
and there may I be alone,
and enter into prayer,
to talk with the One to whom I belong.

May I express there everything in my heart,
and may all the foliage of the field –
all grasses, trees, and plants –
awake at my coming,
to send the powers of their life into the words of my prayer

so that my prayer and speech are made whole
through the life and the spirit of all growing things,
which are made as one by their transcendent Source.

May I then pour out the words of my heart
before your Presence like water, God,
and lift up my hands to You in song,
on my behalf, and that of my children!

Adapted from Likutey Moharan,
Part I, #52 of Reb Nachman of Breslov[37]

Things To Think About And Do

1.   It's your body! Seek information about complementary and alternative health practices to complement your medical treatment.

2.   Explore creative arts to tap into your imagination.

3.   Find a humor coach to lighten your spirit.

4.   Sing while you take a shower or a walk.

5.   Journal your worries and feelings after a difficult experience.

6.   Don't just do something; sit there! Focus on slow breathing to connect with your inner spirit.

7.   Select a mantra, inspirational word, or favorite message to carry with you.

8.   Develop a personal visualization that relaxes or calms you.

9.   Enjoy nature daily and remember to nurture your inner garden.

10. Pull weeds furiously when angry.

11. Reflect on new meaning and purpose: What is your song?

Chapter Twelve

A Treasure Chest Of Traditional And Modern Spiritual Tools

D uring my illness journey I turned to my Jewish tradition for help with coping and renewing my spirit. While all religions have inspiring spiritual practices, my faith and familiarity with Judaism enabled me to enthusiastically explore the virtual treasure chest of resources awaiting me there that can help in situations of illness and injury. The alphabetically-arranged list of traditional and contemporary spiritual tools in this chapter includes prayer, Psalms, rituals and ancestral wisdom, stories and texts, and *tikkun olam*.

> *Prayer may not bring water to parched fields, nor mend a broken bridge, nor rebuild a ruined city. But prayer can water an arid soul, mend a broken heart, and rebuild a weakened will.*
>
> *To pray is to open a door where both God and soul may enter. Prayer is an act which makes the heart audible to God.*
>
> Rabbi Abraham Joshua Heschel

Prayer

The psychological and physiological benefits of prayer have made it the most common unconventional healing practice in America, used by 91% of women and 85% of men.[1] Specific prayers express gratitude and praise, petition for protection from suffering, seek inspiration for endurance, and offer community blessings. According to cardiologist Dr. Mehmet Oz, most patients on his cardiac service consider prayer their only method of complementary medicine.[2] Patients with greater stress and less social support are more likely to turn to God or a Higher Power.

If you wonder, "does prayer really work?" here are some thoughts to consider.[3] Prayer seems to work when what one asks for actually comes about, or when a person senses God's presence in a quiet, peaceful, or inspired state. Repetitive chanting of certain prayers can calm the body and counteract effects of stress. Prayer can distract a person from his or her suffering or enable the person to face discomfort with greater equanimity. Prayer may help people feel less alone and more connected to their religious heritage and community. Prayer can also increase awareness of blessings and develop empathy for those less fortunate.

> *"Where is God to be found? In the place where He is given entry."*
>
> Rabbi Menachem Mendel of Kotsk

While many people use prayer as a coping tool, some find prayer irrelevant or don't believe in God, perhaps having been turned off at an earlier age. Others don't know how to approach prayer or feel uncomfortable with the formal structure of prayer. For those individuals it might be helpful to think of prayer as a search for personal inspiration, whether voiced aloud or silently. We can pray through silence, by humming or daydreaming, and through awareness of our body's rhythms.

Prayer is not only about what you are thinking. You might want to reflect on what you are most concerned about and what emotions you feel the need to express. The most effective prayers are those in which a person asks for inner strengthening because the very act of orienting toward a desired goal often becomes self-fulfilling. The Hebrew word, "*kavannah*" refers to "with intention" or literally, "with a direction."

The most important thing is sincerity and positive intention. The repeated practice of prayer can create a relationship with a higher power the more frequently it is used. It is said that God hears all prayers, even those not spoken, and that God is near to those with a broken heart.

> *"Every human being is tied to God by a rope. If the rope breaks, and is later fixed with a knot, that individual is connected even closer to God than if there never had been a*

break in the rope. Thus, errors, mistakes, and failures have
the potential of drawing us even closer to God."

Hasidic Teaching

In Genesis when God calls to Adam and Eve: "Where Art Thou?" God knows where they are, but is really asking where they are in their lives spiritually. A contemporary view of prayer[4] as an opportunity for self-awareness and emotional vulnerability may particularly appeal to Baby Boomers, who are a "generation of seekers."[5] Here the emphasis shifts from focus on the content of prayer to the experience of being emotionally present.

"Two things are all you really need to know in order to
pray – who you are, and what it is you feel today."

Rabbi Ron Shulman[6]

Prayers voiced in contemporary language may help us feel more connected to our inner spirit. For example, the following prayer seeking rest and renewal might help a person transition from a hectic work week to the beginning of the Sabbath day of rest. It uses language filled with imagery from nature to induce benevolent physiological changes, emotional states, and important life lessons.

A Prayer for Modern Man / Woman

Slow me down, Lord!

Ease the pounding of my heart by the quieting of my mind.

Steady my hurried pace with a vision of the eternal reach of time.

Give me, amidst the confusion of the day,
the calmness of the everlasting hills.

Break the tension of my nerves and muscles with the soothing
music of the singing streams that live in my memory.

Help me to know the magical restorative power of sleep.

Teach me the art of taking minute vacations, of slowing down to
look at a flower, to chat with a friend, to pet a dog, to read a few
lines from a good book.

Remind me each day of the fable of the hare and the tortoise that I may know that the race is not always to the swift; that there is more to life than increasing its speed.

Let me look upward into the branches of the towering trees, and know that they grow tall because they grow slowly and well.

Slow me down, Lord, and inspire me to send my roots deep into the soil of life's enduring values, that I may grow toward the start of my great destiny.

Wilferd Arlan Peterson[7]

Rabbi Abraham Joshua Heschel recommends a daily practice of asking oneself: "What surprised me today?, What inspired me today? What moved me today?" to help us pay attention and appreciate more. He also urges us to translate our discontents into taking steps on behalf of social justice, which he sees as the path to holiness. Rather than asking for something from God, Heschel suggests we think about what God might ask of us.

Heschel describes prayer as a ladder on which to mount our thoughts to God, clarify our hopes and intentions in the world, and become less self-absorbed as we open ourselves to God's presence.

Prayer is a ladder on which our thoughts mount to God.
Prayer takes our mind out of the narrowness of self-interest.
Prayer clarifies our hopes and our intentions.
Prayer, like a gulf stream, imparts warmth to all that is cold.
Prayer is a dialogue with God.
Prayer is an answer to God.
Prayer is an invitation to God to intervene in our lives.
Prayer is our desire to let God's will prevail in our affairs.
Prayer is opening our soul to God.
Prayer is our intention to make God the master of our soul.
Prayer is to sense God's presence.
Prayer is a gift to God.

Rabbi Abraham Joshua Heschel

Judaism has many prayers focusing on gratitude to God for our bodily functioning. A very important body-oriented daily prayer recited by observant Jews after rising and using the bathroom, is *Asher Yatzar* ("Who created"). Composed by Abayei, a Babylonian Rabbi in the 4th century BC, this prayer speaks of the myriad of vessels, channels, and tubes of the body that must either open or close for proper functioning. Reciting it reminds us to not take our bodies for granted, and to recognize that man, unlike animals, has the ability to imbue these functions with higher spiritual consciousness.[8, 9] *Asher Yatzar* is a wonderful, multipurpose prayer that applies to almost every organ system of the body.

Another daily prayer from the morning liturgy is *Elohai Neshama*, which speaks of the Divine breath and spirit implanted in each of us by God. This prayer complements *Asher Yatzar* in its focus on the body. When healthy, we take in oxygen and exhale carbon dioxide effortlessly, but for those with lung conditions, it is a more difficult effort. This prayer reminds us that the God-given Divine breath and spark in each of us must be lovingly nurtured. The prayer begins as follows:

> *Elohai neshama shenatata bee tehora hee. Atah beratah, atah yetzarta, atah nefakhta bee, v'atah meshamrah bekeerbee. – My God, the soul which You have given me is pure. You created it, You formed it, You breathed it into me. You keep body and soul together.*
>
> Morning liturgy, Siddur[10]

In addition to formal prayers in the *Siddur*, Judaism has a tradition of personal prayers. The very first prayer in the Bible, cried out by Moses when his sister Miriam was struck with leprosy was: *"El na refa na la"* ("Please God, heal her, please"). The brevity and directness of this prayer adds to its emotional intensity. Perhaps this precedent of personal prayer might inspire you to write an original prayer, print it on a "healing card," and carry it with you. As an example, Rabbi Jim Michaels has shared a personal prayer for healing as follows:[11]

Making Your Own "Healing Card"

A Prayer for Healing

In my illness, Lord, I turn to You, for I am your creation.
Your strength and courage are in my spirit,
And Your powers of healing are within my body.
May it be Your will to restore me to health.

In my illness I have learned what is great and what is small.
I know how dependent I am upon You.
My own pain and anxiety have been my teachers.
May I never forget this precious knowledge when I am well again.

Heal me, Lord and I shall be healed, save me and I shall be saved.
Comfort me, Lord, and shelter me in Your love.

Blessed are You, Lord, the faithful and merciful Healer.
Amen.

Ill patients often have difficulty falling and staying asleep at night. When lying still they are more aware of bodily discomforts that make them anxious.

According to a *Midrash*, each night God takes back our soul and returns it in the morning. The *Hashkivenu* prayer in the siddur is like a nightly meditation seeking God's sheltering protection as we sleep, and God's compassionate renewal of our bodies and spirits as we wake each morning. The prayer uses soothing images such as "*sukkat shelomecha*" (your sukkah of peace) and "*kanfei Shekhinah*" (in the shadow of God's wings) to help people feel greater safety, comfort, and hope as we journey through life.

This traditional prayer seeks protection and renewal using soothing images of God's sheltering presence.

Hashkivenu

Hashkivenu Avinu L'Shalom
Our Father, let us lie down in peace
raise us up, our King, to life and peace.

Ufros Aleinu Sukkat Shlomecha
Spread over us the shelter of Your peace.
Guide us with Your good counsel
and deliver us for the sake of Your Name.

Ushmor Tzeitenu U'vo'einu
Safeguard our going and coming
for life and for peace
from now and for all time.

Evening Liturgy, Siddur

Naomi Levy has written a beautiful collection of contemporary personal prayers that resemble intimate conversations with God.[12] Using simple and direct language, many of the prayers seek God's comforting presence to help people feel more protected and less alone when dealing with illness, disability, and life's difficulties.

Prayers seeking protection from suffering, oppression, and loneliness are found in many other religious traditions as well. A Catholic friend gave me a beautiful ancient prayer in which the Virgin Mary appears to the elderly Indian Juan Diego. The prayer contains images of protection and soothing with the powerful message: I am here for you.

Since community is so important in Judaism, many prayers are voiced in the plural and are recited communally, such as *"Refa-eynu"* ("Heal us") and the *"Mi Sheberach"* ("Who that blesses"). The latter is recited during the Torah reading service on behalf of ill members in the congregation. The ill person's mother's Hebrew name is mentioned because God's quality of compassion, called *"rachamim,"* comes from the root *"rechem,"* meaning womb, thus suggesting a mother's care.

Mi Sheberach

May He who blessed our ancestors, Abraham, Isaac, and Jacob, Sara, Rebecca, Rachel, and Leah, bless and heal _____ (person's Hebrew name, followed by mother's Hebrew name).

May the Holy One in mercy strengthen him/her and heal him/her soon, body and soul, together with others who suffer illness. And let us say Amen.

Morning liturgy, Siddur

The *Mi Sheberach* prayer seeks a full healing of body and spirit, yet there are times when patients face oppressive and insurmountable situations, such as in deteriorating or terminal illness. At such times patients need to feel they are not alone in their suffering, as illustrated in this anonymous contemporary prayer:

> *Grant me, O God, the strength to face each hour of this and every day. In fact, when it seems that I cannot face even this hour, please fill me with sufficient strength to face the next five minutes. Amen.*

Jewish tradition also has prayers expressing thanksgiving for reaching a special milestone ("*Shehecheyanu*") or recently surviving a crisis, operation, accident, or near disaster. For the latter, the person comes to synagogue as soon as physically able to following recovery, and offers the *Bircat Hagomel* ("*Benching gomel*") prayer thanking God, which is followed by the congregation's responsive blessing. As important as the individual's public expression of gratitude is the community's welcoming the person back into its midst.

Family caregivers ministering to a sick relative face challenges that are physically and emotionally draining. They could use support because they are engaged in a marathon, not just a sprint. They need to pace themselves and seek adequate rest alongside their efforts, advice that is easier said than done. The following is a prayer that can be recited by caregivers:

A Prayer For Caregivers To Say

Dear God, source of light and inspiration,
Thank you for entrusting me with the task and opportunity to
do caregiving.
Please give me patience and strength to offer compassion and an
open heart to those who suffer.
May you bless those who need care with your Divine love and
healing.
May you grant me wisdom to be aware of my needs and nurture
myself through self-care, so that I can better serve those in need.

Israela Meyerstein

Psalms

Psalms have been recited since ancient times to comfort people facing illness, suffering, and hardship. King David is credited with having authored Psalms while he was fleeing for his life and being hunted by King Saul.

Today there are *"tehillim"* groups that gather to recite Psalms on behalf of patients' well-being. Whether intercessory prayer works remains controversial,[13] but certainly patients feel comforted knowing that others are keeping them in thoughts and prayers.

Saturated with intense emotion, varying moods, and dramatic language, Psalms have appeal because they help people feel understood by mirroring moods that patients experience, such as sadness, fear, despair, hope, and gratitude. Psalms describing human struggles against odds can strengthen patients' resolve to persevere.

Psalms are addressed to a Higher Power and often pose challenging spiritual questions. Originally written in Hebrew and translated into Old English, the language may feel antiquated to some. There are, however, excellent and more accessible contemporary books of Psalms for the modern reader such as those by Steven Mitchell, Danny Siegel, and Debbie Perlman.

Reb Nachman of Breslov identified certain "healing" Psalms as part of a "comprehensive remedy," or *"Tikkun Klali,"* that he believed could uplift the mind, rectify one's failures, and cleanse the soul (Psalms 16, 32, 41, 42, 59, 77, 90, 105, 137, 150). Each Psalm has a different tone. For example, Psalm 16 reflects an ill person seeking God's support; Psalm 32 anticipates recovery, and Psalm 41 is a meditation on suffering.[14]

Perhaps the most universally recited Psalm is the 23rd Psalm. Written in beautiful Hebrew and English poetry, it gives thanks and petitions God's presence to help humans endure struggles and not feel alone or afraid. In our spiritual study/discussion groups we offered "Psalm clips" (fragments of Psalms on slips of paper) to group members and asked them to select one that personally resonated with their circumstances.

One elderly woman selected the line from Psalm 23, "though I walk through the valley of the shadow of death" and related it to a situation of upcoming surgery. She described how instead of focusing on her fears, she courageously "walked" into the surgical room to face her procedure. We encouraged participants to keep the Psalm clip in their pocket or wallet for use as needed.

The following Psalm speaks to the constraints imposed by illness.

> *"Min hamaytzar karati yah, ana-nee bamerchavya – Out of the narrow place, I call to You, God. Answer me with Your expansiveness."*
>
> Psalm 118

The Psalm begins with a play on words describing the narrowness of illness and likening it to the "narrow straits" (*"maytzar"*) of Egypt (*"Mitzrayim"*) during slavery. The Psalmist seeks God's help in finding options and a wider perspective. I have used this Psalm when grappling with personal challenges and to help patients deal with difficult people and situations in their lives. Reciting or singing the Psalm creates enough of a pause to reflect and be less over-reactive. By remembering strengths that helped me handle past stressful situations I am often able to respond with more flexibility and confidence.

One of my favorite Psalms is Psalm 90:

> *"Teach us to number our days that we may acquire a heart of wisdom."*

Psalms help us cope with our transient nature in the universe by reminding us to make meaningful use of our time. For people who are ill and whose time is limited, this Psalm might motivate them to make the most of their precious remaining time.

Rituals And Ancestral Wisdom

"When words are inadequate, have a ritual."

Anonymous

Rituals have been a part of religion, culture, and healing ceremonies for centuries. Referred to as humankind's original form of therapy, spiritually-based rituals symbolize important moments and transitions in people's lives, and can be effective coping strategies for handling stressful life events.[15] Rituals are powerful behavioral practices because of their ability to represent and intensify emotional experience.

Many rituals are time-bound, lending tradition and structure to daily life. They involve the intentional repetition of words, music, food, drinks, smells, sights, ceremony, and behavior to mark continuity and transition.[16] Examples are family meals and life cycle events in community. Some rituals mark transitions from one state to another, such as the *Havdalah* ceremony on Saturday night to demarcate the sacred Sabbath from the start of the new secular work week.

Judaism has many rituals that embody traditional values such as resting on the Sabbath, which symbolizes God's resting on the seventh day after creation. The Sabbath ritual slows down our fast-paced lives and carves out time for reflection, family, and community worship. The *mikveh* (ritual bath) marks a transition between the unclean and the clean. Originally intended for women upon completion of their menstrual period to indicate they are ready for sexual relations, it is also used by young men and women (separately) before their wedding to mark the sacred transition between single and married life. The *mikveh* has also been used as a therapeutic ritual to help a person feel cleansed after healing from abuse, trauma, or illness.

Rituals can also mark important calendar events such as the lighting of a *Yahrzheit* (memorial) candle to remember one's deceased relatives on the anniversary of their death. When my mother was within weeks of dying, I organized a 40th anniversary wedding celebration with immediate family, marking it with an anniversary cake, a calligraphed *ketubah* (wedding certificate) whose text was surrounded by a collage of pictures chronicling their lives together. While a bittersweet occasion, lovingly designing the *ketubah* was therapeutic for me and helped us all prepare for endings. I know it was meaningful for my parents to see a reflection of all they had accomplished together in life.

Rituals can also help patients undergoing illness and treatment. The Radiation Unit at Johns Hopkins Medical Center has a powerful ritual for patients when they complete their final radiation treatment.[17] The following poem is read, and then the patient energetically bangs a gong. Relatives and friends come to share cake and take pictures of the event signifying an end to treatment and a fresh beginning:

"Your day has come to strike the bell
Your silent heart has much to tell
And much to toll this proud new day
Treatment done, you're on your way."

Mary Kathleen Adcock, Radiation patient

My friend's daughter had just finished a horrendous year of chemotherapy for Lymphoma, remission, recurrence, a bone marrow transplant, and radiation. She proclaimed: "I feel like it's ringing in a New Year – a fresh start – a time for health and happiness." Her mother read a long emotional poem about the family's ordeal that left not a single dry eye in the room.

You can create your own meaningful rituals to symbolize important transitions. During treatment my husband and I planned a vacation so that we could look forward to something joyous once I felt well enough. Upon completing treatment I recited the *"Shehecheyanu"* prayer, celebrating having reached that important milestone. On my 60th birthday I traded in my gas-guzzling SUV for a new car in "fire engine red" that I named "spirit" to symbolize my new-found zest in life.

Traditional rituals can also be given new meanings. For example, before the Passover holiday, a preparatory ritual involves cleaning and ridding the house of *"chametz,"* or leavened products. Expanding the definition of *"chametz"* to include emotional baggage, such as non-constructive thoughts, behaviors, and harmful habits can deepen the ritual's meaning. Letting go of pieces of "emotional *chametz*" can make Passover a time of spiritual cleansing as well.

Ancestral Wisdom

In our growing up years my sisters and I witnessed our parents and their siblings performing the ritual of visiting graves of departed family members before the High Holidays. This ritual of generational continuity pays respect to ancestors. We, the visitors, turn to them to ask for blessings for the coming year based on the belief that ancestors are closer to God, and can intercede on behalf of the living.

As young adults we dutifully accompanied our elderly aunt out of respect, but winced privately as she "spoke" to our dead parents, sister, and grandmother. After my aunt died, however, we found ourselves continuing the tradition of "graveside chats" each year by reading her letters, writing our own, and discussing family stories and values. Sometimes these visits included spouses and even children; perhaps our children also wince, but meanwhile they are learning about generational continuity.

During my year of illness and treatment, the cemetery visit felt both more unsettling as well as more spiritual. I recited a letter of gratitude for surviving and asked for my parents to continue watching over me and my family. As I stood at my parents' graves and closed my eyes, I visualized their kindly presence and felt their comforting love, as if reaching across some impenetrable barrier.

"The Spirit is mightier than the grave."
Rabbi Maurice Lamm

Cemeteries are not typically thought of as places of choice for family gatherings except when necessary, but in other cultures a stronger relationship exists between the living and the dead.

> *"You yourself are the embodied continuance of those who did not live in your time and others will be (and are) your continuity on earth..."*
>
> Jorge Luis Borges, cited in
> M. McGoldrick, *The Legacy of Loss*

Thornton Wilder in the Bridge of San Luis Rey, offers comfort when missing a beloved person:

> *"There is a land of the living and a land of the dead and the bridge is love, the only survival, the only meaning."*

My sisters and I plan to continue our "graveside chats" as long as we are physically able to because these visits create an outlet to express appreciation for our parents' lives. It is also an opportunity to reflect on how their values and ideals continue to inspire us in the present. Visiting gravesites is a privilege unique to my generation as my parents and husband's parents had no graves to visit because their immediate relatives were gassed in concentration camps during the Holocaust. I feel that the task of transmitting this ritual to the next generation is a spiritual and moral imperative.

> *"Death ends a life but not a relationship."*
>
> Robert Anderson
> *I Never Sang for My Father*

Stories And Texts

> *"Telling stories takes us further along the road to wholeness and healing."*
>
> Blanchard[18]

Stories, whether oral or written, can enchant us while teaching important life lessons and serving as inspirational guides for overcoming challenges. Stories can be complex, multilayered, and tap into deeper parts of ourselves. They can help us accept our limitations and learn from mistakes. Great storytellers such as Elie Wiesel used his stories to figuratively blow a *shofar* to wake us up about important events and experience.

Narratives within religious traditions interpret ancient texts about struggles to overcome challenges as an opportunity to transmit lessons for future generations. A quintessential example is the Passover *Haggadah*, a text recited annually at the Passover Seder, which inspires Jews of all ages to remember their people's roots, survival stories, and values. Biblical stories contain symbols of transformation, such as the story of Jacob, perhaps the first "wounded healer." After wrestling with an angel and being injured, Jacob's name was changed to Israel and he was promised that he would father a great people.

The Talmud contains an exhaustive collection of rabbinic debates and discussions offering detailed views about coping with illness, treatment of the sick, and visitation guidelines that still inform our practices today. For example, when the Rabbis urge "sweeping the floor" in the patient's room, they are using a metaphor for inspection of the patient's physical surroundings to assure the patient's physical comfort. One Rabbinic story reminds us that even in the presence of good friends, a patient may experience a range of difficult emotions under the surface. They therefore remind us of the importance of letting the patient guide visitors as to what he or she needs.

End of life issues are beautifully illustrated in the Talmudic story about the death of Rabbi Judah the Prince.[19] In this story, the Rabbi is near death and in a lot of physical pain. His devoted students, however, continue to pray for his miraculous recovery because they rely on him. The Rabbi's handmaiden, who is sensitive to the Rabbi's suffering, takes matters into her own hands by throwing down a jar from the roof of the Rabbi's house and uttering a prayer. In that brief moment when the noise of the jar breaking distracts the students from praying, the Rabbi's soul is freed from his suffering and he dies.

Not infrequently a patient hangs on to life by a thread, unable to die until family members "give permission" to let go. I have used this story with friends in such situations and have witnessed its powerful effect on the "letting go" process of a dying relative.

Hasidic tales and parables tell about life wounds and regrettable choices to help readers reflect, learn, and grow from mistakes. Stories tap into parts of us that may be below consciousness and can show us a mirror of ourselves to help us face vulnerabilities, accept our failings, and heal. One of my favorite stories is about developing a perspective on the ups and downs of life.

This Too Shall Pass

A man who is undergoing great troubles in his life goes to a wise craftsman for relief of his woes. The craftsman shows the man a very special ring, allegedly handed down from the great and wise King Solomon. On the ring is inscribed the phrase *"gam zeh ya'avor."* (This too shall pass). The man queries the meaning of the words, and is pleased when told that his bad luck and troubles will soon pass. The man wears the ring every day and indeed his life does turn around. He is so delighted that he returns to thank the craftsman for his new-found blessings and riches and to seek more wonderful news. He asks the craftsman what other predictions for his future the magic ring portends. The craftsman smiles wisely, and again states the ring's message: "This too shall pass."

This story reminds us of life's hills and valleys over which we have no control. Sometimes hoping and expecting life to be all positive inadequately prepares us for dealing with hardship. Buddhist wisdom teaches that suffering is a natural part of life that can, at times, teach us important lessons. Put differently, we must cherish our blessings and also learn to accept times of hardship and struggle.

Stories can teach us to face life's difficulties and emerge stronger in spirit. In one story, a Rabbi directs a newly-widowed woman who is bitterly complaining about her suffering, to search for people who do not know suffering. In returning empty-handed she learns that loss is part of human life and that she is not being singled out. Moreover, by reaching out to other people in her search, she comes to accept comfort from others. Another story, *The Wagon Bears the Burden,*[20] encourages patients and caregivers to learn to accept help.

Stories can delight us, puzzle us, and teach us to mine valuable lessons to apply to our own lives. One of my favorite stories has always been "The Little Engine That Could," about a train that needed to find courage and self-confidence to solve a problem. It is a story that I have used to motivate myself, my children, and even clients where applicable.

Patients and caregivers can find a treasure trove of contemporary stories on the internet about facing stress and adversity, accepting limitations, healing, and thriving. For example, one story called *Stillness* tells about a wounded bird's need for "stillness" to heal from within.[21] Another about *"A Carrot, an Egg, and a Cup of Coffee"*[22] reminds us of our freedom to choose our response to challenges.

Tikkun Olam

"Living is not a private affair of the individual. Living is what man does with God's time, what man does with God's world."

Abraham Joshua Heschel

Illness and injury rob us of strength and force us to lean on and accept help from others. If we are able to get out, participating in a support group can connect us to a caring community. If we do not have the strength to go out, internet support sites and chat rooms offer alternative ways of connecting with others. When we recover sufficiently, we can repay kindnesses by reaching out to help others. Looking for meaningful, if only small, ways to lift their spirits can give us renewed sense of purpose as well. Acts that bring light, holiness, and healing into the world are the essence of *"tikkun olam,"* one of the more powerful spiritual coping tools.

"The best way to find yourself is to lose yourself in the service of others."

Gandhi

While the phrase *"tikkun olam"* (repair of the world) originated as early as the *Mishnaic* period (200 CE), a more contemporary meaning comes from the teachings of the 16th century mystic and Kabbalist, Rabbi Isaac Luria.[23] In the Lurianic view, God contracted himself into vessels to create the world and then the vessels shattered. It was left up to man to collect the scattered holy sparks.

This belief represented a theological change reflecting God's search for man as a partner in repairing the world. Though the term *"tikkun olam"* disappeared after the 16th century, it re-emerged in the late 20th century when American Jewish cultural values co-opted the term in response to evolving political and social developments. *Tikkun olam* can also include showing kindness in day-to-day interactions.

> *"No act of kindness, no matter how small, is ever wasted."*
>
> Aesop

Danny Siegel devoted his career to inspiring and encouraging people to perform deeds of service for those less fortunate. Through his foundation, he funded projects he called "Mitzvah therapy"[24] to provide outlets for service and charitable giving. In Judaism, performing a *"mitzvah"* or good deed, is of great importance. It is said that giving charity and repenting can bring Divine forgiveness and personal healing. Studies show that acting altruistically by helping others lowers stress and impacts positively on the giver's spirit and well-being.[25]

> *"If you want to feel united with God, stop talking and do a mitzvah, any mitzvah."*
>
> Solomon Schechter

Bill O'Hanlon identifies *mitzvah* therapy as an important spiritual pathway.[26] He relates the well-known Ericksonian story of the "violet lady," a solitary woman suffering from loneliness and an intractable, medication-resistant depression, whose only pleasure was solo gardening. Erickson, a master hypnotist, convinced her to begin a practice of delivering her violet plant cuttings to people in the community. She begrudgingly began doing this and continued the practice for many years. When she died in old age, hundreds of grateful people came to show their appreciation. The above story shows that just taking steps to initiate an activity can eventually lead to an unexpectedly positive outcome.

A chronically ill patient wrote a book about how doing one kind deed a day can lead to a more positive outlook, less self-involvement, and more connection to others.[27] Several long term studies found that volunteering can even make a difference in staying alive.[28] As volunteers, we often experience good feelings and a "helper's high" when we give. When I do something that lifts the spirits of a sick friend, I am touched by how this gesture makes my day. Doing good deeds is a spiritual uplift that adds meaning to life and emulates Divine qualities. The giver always receives at least as much as he or she gives.

The following is a beautiful inspirational reading for those interested in *tikkun olam*.

Courage

You dare to call us partners;
We will live, one day at a time,
performing signs and wonders for the benefit of others.
This we promise you.

You dare to call us little lower than the angels;
We will use our face and hands to be Your messengers.
To this we commit ourselves this day.

You dare to tell us that we are fashioned in Your image;
We will be this Image, live our lives
by the most Divine in us,
and in this Image listen to Your words and do Your will.
So we solemnly declare this day.

Your Mitzvah opportunities await.
*Give us strength: We vow to do Your will
as, by Your light and guidance,
our hearts and souls so move us.*

Danny Siegel[29]

Things To Think About And Do

1. What concerns and yearnings do you feel a need to express?

2. What is your preferred way of praying?

3. Write a personal prayer on a card to carry with you.

4. Select a meaningful Psalm clip to keep with you.

5. What coping tools do you use for fears at night?

6. Reflect on which rituals are most meaningful to you or create one.

7. Set aside one day a week for rest, reflection, and time with family.

8. Tap into the power of stories; make a time and place in your week for reading.

9. Connect with a community for support, friendship, and or religious fellowship.

10. If you are a caregiver, how do you recharge your batteries?

11. When you are able, consider even small ways of giving back and helping others.

12. What connects you with those ancestors who came before?

13. How do you understand "death does not defeat life?"

PART IV
GUIDED REFLECTIONS
AND
EXERCISES FOR COPING
AND HEALING

Chapter Thirteen

Personal Spiritual Self-Assessment

W hat is a Spiritual Assessment? In Judaism, the ancient practice of *"Bikur Cholim"* was viewed as a kind of assessment of how the patient was doing. The word *"bikur"* literally means "visit, search after, delve into" the patient's physical condition, mental disposition, spiritual attitude and needs. By checking into our emotional state, we can better understand how illness has affected our bodies and souls.

Spirituality seeks to make meaning out of crisis. It helps us look inwardly to reflect on our current responses to illness and identify pathways for healing. Existential questions may help you focus on how you respond to struggles of existence.[1] How would you answer the following existential questions?

- **How** are you managing with the challenges you are facing?
- **How** has illness affected you and your family?
- **Where** do you turn for comfort?
- **What** gives you strength, courage, and inspiration to go on?
- **When** your spirits are low, who or what lifts you up?
- **Who** provides support, companionship, or assistance?
- **What** do you need right now?

Spirituality is expressed outwardly through different pathways (community, religion) and inwardly by connecting with one's inner spirit, or Divine spark. Being "in touch" with ourselves is central to the process of inner connection and healing. A spiritual assessment begins with an emotional self-evaluation reflecting on feelings commonly experienced.

As you review the list of feelings that follow, which ones are current emotions or states you frequently experience? You may want to make a list of those that are relevant to you. What do you notice about the adjectives you selected? Which feelings are the most difficult for you? Which emotions have you experienced when facing personal illness, crisis, or trauma in yourself or a family member or loved one?

Assessing Emotional States

Abandoned
Abused
Aimless
Alone
Angry   Disillusioned
Anxious   Downhearted
Betrayed   Empty
Bitter   Enslaved
Blamed   Excited   Invisible
Blessed   Exhausted   Irritable
Burdened   Fearful   Isolated
Calm   Fragile   Joyful
Comforted   Frantic   Lost   Stable
Competent   Frustrated   Loved   Strong
Confused   Gloomy   Misunderstood   Stupid
Content   Grateful   Neglected   Supported
Defeated   Guilty   Nurtured   Terrified
Depressed   Helpless   Overwhelmed   Threatened
Determined   Hopeful   Panicky   Trapped
                 Impatient   Pessimistic   Trusting
                 Incompetent   Protected   Unappreciated
                 Insecure   Resentful   Unsafe
                 Inspired   Responsible   Upset
                                  Sad   Unsupported
                                  Secure   Weak
                                  Sensitive   Weary
                                  Spirited   Withdrawn
                                                   Worried
                                                   Wounded

State Of The Spirit

In his spiritual counseling, Rabbi Simkha Weintraub developed a "State of the Spirit"[2] to help individuals frame their experience of self in the world. While not quantifiable, a "state of the spirit" is a qualitative assessment that reveals how a person views himself or herself emotionally and spiritually. Rabbi Weintraub lists 36 state of the spirit descriptives, of which several contrasting states are represented below.

- Vulnerable and exposed vs. strengthened and shielded
- Despairing and hopeless vs. hopeful and trusting
- Bitter and sad vs. joyful and content
- Disconnected and lonely vs. connected and communal
- Reactive and rigid vs. responsive and flexible
- Meaningless and empty vs. purposeful and fulfilled
- Fearful and avoidant vs. courageous and responsible
- Overwhelmed and cornered vs. inspired and expansive

In reviewing the above list of contrasting states, which of each pair seems to resonate more? Does your self-description tell you something about the state of your spirit?

The following general questions explore your current spiritual connections to community, a higher power, and/or spiritual beliefs and practices. These questions are adapted from Jewish Family Services Spiritual Assessment by Weintraub, Asking About Spirituality (Weintraub),[3] and the Joint Commission on Accreditation of Health Organizations,[4] which now mandates exploration of spirituality in counseling.

Spirituality/Religion As A Resource In Daily Life

1. How would you identify your own spiritual/religious heritage? How do you express it?
2. Do you belong to a church, synagogue, mosque, ashram, meeting house, or other place of worship?
3. Do you have a relationship with a clergy person or spiritual guide?

4. Do you feel a connection, however remote or latent, to a spiritual community?
5. Do you turn to God or some other higher power as a source of comfort? Did you ever?
6. When experiencing distress or pain, do you derive comfort from any religious beliefs, spiritual practices, or sacred writings? If so, how do these help you?

Spiritual Assessment also asks us to reflect on where we came from, where we are now, and where we are going. Spiritual roots are about family remembrances since it is in our families where identity, values, and life attitudes are forged. Reflecting on origins of our spiritual beliefs, practices, and connections can deepen our understanding of how early childhood spiritual lessons and experiences have impacted our current attitudes to spirituality.

Guided Remembering encourages us to reflect on those experiences, both positive and negative, that have meaning for us. For example, memories of attending services with a beloved grandparent can evoke feelings of love and comfort. By contrast, painful memories of harsh family conflicts over differences in belief and practice may have led to distancing and disconnection. Trauma experienced in conjunction with religious experience may continue to cast a shadow on current attitudes and relationships. Reviewing and reappraising these past influences can open the possibility of coming to terms with them or making new spiritual connections. The following excerpted questions are adapted from a more thorough spiritual history assessment by Janine Roberts.[5]

Spiritual History Assessment

1. What is your first memory of what you would call a spiritual or religious encounter? How did it affect you?
2. What was passed down through the generations to you about religious and/or spiritual beliefs and values?
3. What life cycle rituals, ceremonies were observed in your family? What values did you learn from these practices?
4. Who taught and most influenced you about spiritual/ religious beliefs as a child?

5. What gender messages did you absorb about yourself as a boy or girl through spiritual/religious activities, beliefs, experiences?
6. How did family members use or not use religious/spiritual beliefs and practices to get through difficult times? Did changes occur in family spiritual/religious practices over time?
7. How have your identities (as a single or partnered person, divorced, gay, heterosexual, transgender, a person who has physical, mental, or other challenges, parent, etc.) been supported or not supported by religious or traditional doctrine? Where do you get support for your identities?

After reflecting on these questions, what feelings or insights do you have about the influence of earlier spiritual/religious experiences on who you are today?

Spiritual Evaluation

Additional questions to explore spiritual connections, as part of self-assessment, might be:

1. What would you say is your key "lament?"[6] What induces in you the strongest worry, upset, fear, or suffering? What is your biggest "Oy?"
2. Do you think you have mild concerns, moderate distress, or severe despair?[7]
3. Do you connect with something bigger outside yourself: with people, community, nature, or other spiritual pathways?[8]

If we can find meaning in our troubles that renews our spirit and purpose, our search will have been worthwhile. Reflecting on the following questions may be therapeutic in itself.

1. How do you make sense of your present crisis situation?
2. What matters most to you? Do you have spiritual goals?
3. What do you need to renew your spirit?
4. What strengths have you used in the past to cope with adversity?
5. Are there difficult feelings, disappointments, and questions that remain with you?

Chapter Fourteen

Journey Of Life Exercise

T he Journey of Life or *Darchei Chayim* exercise, developed by my colleague Rabbi Gila Ruskin and me,[1] was inspired by the work of Peter Steinglass[2] with families facing chronic illness. This exercise will help you reflect on your unique strengths, examine the impact of your illness experience, and seek spiritual coping tools to help you move in a healing direction.

The "Illness Journey" is likened to the travels of the ancient Israelites wandering in the wilderness after leaving Egypt. They journeyed for forty years in foreign, unfamiliar territory that was fraught with uncertainty, danger, and vulnerability. As a nation, and as individuals, the people sought comfort and direction, while trying to develop internal and communal survival resources to transcend the wilderness experience.

This creative exercise involves reflection, writing, and some drawing if desired. You can use colored pencils, crayons, markers, or pens to describe your experience. The chart that follows illustrates a three-part journey:

1. Your unique identity, valued strengths, or Divine spark.
2. The detour and emotional impact caused by the illness or crisis.
3. Selecting coping tools for comfort, support, and inspiration to get you through the difficult wilderness and on the path towards healing.
4. Pathways to healing.

Your Unique Identity
Divine Spark / Inner Strengths

Please begin by looking at the chart, starting with (1) at the left.

Begin by focusing on your breathing, something we do naturally and continuously, almost without awareness. Try to

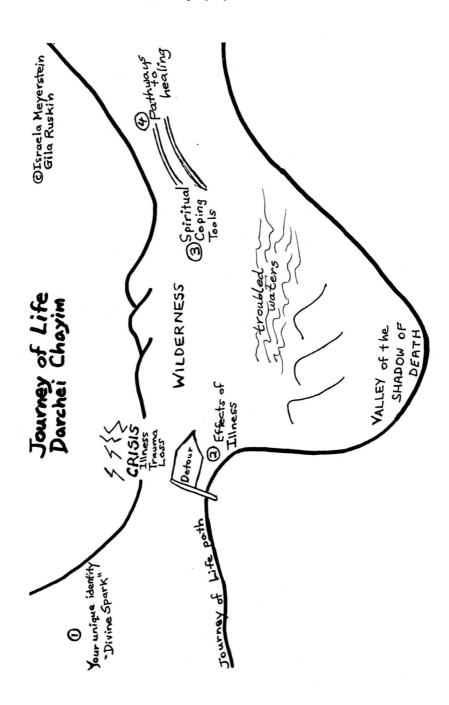

Journey of Life
Darchei Chayim

©Israela Meyerstein
Gila Ruskin

① Your unique identity "Divine Spark"

CRISIS
Illness
Trauma
Loss

Detour

② Effects of Illness

WILDERNESS

③ Spiritual Coping Tools

④ Pathways to healing

troubled waters

VALLEY of the SHADOW of DEATH

Journey of Life path

concentrate on your breath going in and out. As you breathe, you might reflect on the gifts of breath and spirit implanted within you, along with your "Divine spark" that makes you unique. Like a set of fingerprints, no two individuals are alike.

The Divine spark, planted at birth, makes you who you are. It cannot be taken away, even when adversity such as illness, trauma, loss, and addiction diminish the spark, clouds our perspective, and dampens our confidence and hope. Connecting with and nourishing our inner spark can reactivate it to shine brighter and emanate from us.[3] Try to reflect on your unique special qualities and valued strengths.

(For the next exercise, you are permitted to make a photocopy of the chart for your personal use, in order to complete the activity. Do not write in the book if it is not your copy. No other use of the chart is permitted without written permission from the Publisher.)

Next to (1) write some descriptive words or draw symbols, colors, or designs to describe or represent your Divine spark, your special traits and uniqueness in the world.

Current Crisis And Detour Into Wilderness

Imagine you are walking along the familiar winding path of your life at your own comfortable pace. Occasional signposts have helped you anticipate bumps in the road such that you know where to turn. While at times you have encountered challenges that have made life more difficult, over time, you have developed your own pace. You may even feel grateful for the familiarity of the journey.

Suddenly, as you walk, stroll, jog, or race, unexpected ominous clouds signal a dangerous storm immediately ahead. You're alarmed because there's not enough time to get out of harm's way. The crisis could be sudden injury, illness, loss, or trauma. You discover that your immediate path is blocked and you are forced to take a long unexpected detour through a foreign land ... perhaps a hospital, with its confusing procedures, administered by strangers speaking a language you barely understand.

These new surroundings feel like an uncharted path in a

wilderness without signposts and you have no map, GPS, or iPhone. There are high mountains, deep valleys, and unexpected curves in the road. You may even stumble into the Valley of the Shadow of Death. You cannot turn back and are unsure how long this detour in your life will take, or how to get back to your familiar lifepath. Your old maps for coping don't work, thus leaving you feeling vulnerable, uncertain, and alone. Like the ancient Israelites, you may feel frustration, anxiety about surviving, and even experience a crisis of faith. You don't know where to find comfort, support, and strength to weather the rest of the difficult journey.

Can you describe the current crisis situation you are facing and how it is affecting you? What feelings are evoked?

Next to (2) write some words or draw pictures, symbols, or colors to portray your feelings about being in the wilderness of illness and how your spirit has been impacted.

Spiritual Survival Tools For The Wilderness

What helped the ancient Israelites survive in the wilderness? The people embraced a spiritual faith relationship with God and were sustained by Moses' leadership, signs of Divine protection along the way, and their growth as a community. According to the Bible, God provided a pillar of cloud and a pillar of fire as signposts along the way for inspiration, guidance, and protection. Portions of manna appeared daily to provide sustenance, and lend hope and confidence for the future.

Take a moment to reflect on your current situation. Before problem solving, one must first identify feelings and needs. For some people, even having needs may be a foreign concept. By giving yourself permission to reflect, perhaps you will discover needs you never knew existed. Ask yourself:

- What do I need now?

- What are some coping tools you know of that might help you now?

- What personal strengths do you remember calling upon in previous situations of difficulty?

- Reflect on prior coping mechanisms that provided comfort and strengthening.

Key For Journey Of Life:
Biblical Symbols As Spiritual Coping Tools

Look at these Biblical pictographs. Feel free to draw your version of these symbols or create other symbols.

The various symbols from Biblical and religious tradition offer inspiration, guidance, wisdom, and comfort. Some symbols, such as the Burning Bush, refer to experiences in which individuals were inspired by Divine connection. Others, like the rainbow, represent a hopeful sign or covenant with God. The Ten Commandments represent learning rules and values that govern our lives. Additional symbols from Jewish tradition are the Ner Tamid, symbolizing light and continuity, and the Shofar, that wake us up to important realities through musical sounds.

- Which of the Biblical symbols, practical spiritual tools, and Jewish resources shared in previous chapters could be of help to you now?
- Do you have your own creative strategies to use on your illness journey on route to healing?

These may be some of the ingredients of your Spiritual Treatment Plan.

Sign (Hope)
I set My **rainbow** in the cloud, and it shall be for a sign of a covenant between Me and the earth. *Genesis 9:13*

Nourishing Source Of Wisdom (Tradition)
Her ways are ways of pleasantness, and all her paths are peace. She is a **tree of life** to those who lay hold on her; and happy is every one who holds her fast. *Proverbs 3: 17-18*

Revelation (Inspiration)
And the Angel of the Lord appeared to him in a flame of fire out of the midst of a bush; and he looked, behold, the **bush burned** with fire, and the bush was not consumed. *Exodus 3:2*

Comfort ("Being With")

The Lord is my shepherd, I shall not want. He makes me lie down in **green pastures** (nature). He leads me beside the **still waters** to restore my soul. He guides me on the right path, for His name's sake. Though I walk through the valley of the shadow of death I shall fear no evil for You are with me. Your **rod and staff** shall comfort me. You prepare a table before me in the presence of my enemies. You anoint my head with oil. **My cup** runs over (gratitude). Surely goodness and mercy shall pursue me all the days of my life and I shall dwell in the **house of the Lord** forever. *Psalms 23*

Angels accompanying me (Dreams, Wrestling, Transformation)

And **Jacob** dreamed, and behold a **ladder** set up on the earth, and the top of it reached to heaven; and behold the angels of God ascending and descending on it. *Genesis 28:12*

Guidance (Direction)

And the Lord went before them by day in **a pillar of cloud**, to lead them the way; and by night in a **pillar of fire** to give them light; to go by day and night. *Exodus 13:21*

Miracles (Faith)

Lift up your rod, and stretch out your hand over the sea and divide it; and the people of Israel shall go on dry ground through the midst of the **Red Sea**. *Exodus 14:6*

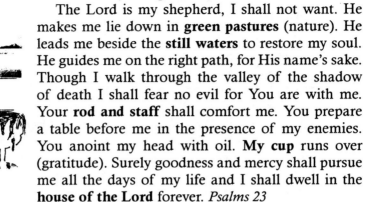

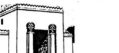

Shelter, Community	Ner Tamid Eternal Light	Torah Learning And Values	Divine Inner Spark

Pathways To Healing

Following is a sample Journey of Life map that I drew using words, symbols, and pictures to represent my experiences. The metaphor of the bridge over troubled waters resonated strongly with me as I tried to use spiritual coping tools to emerge from illness, renew my spirit, and find new pathways for healing.

On your Journey of Life exercise:

- What will your bridge consist of?

- What tools or pathways did you select?

- How did connecting with a Biblical tradition affect you?

- Did you find relevance in ancient traditional resources, or did you develop your own resources to sustain your spirits and preserve identity in the face of illness?

- Which tools increased your sense of agency and connection?

- What did you learn about yourself through this ordeal?

- Did you find some new meaningful pathways?

I hope that the *Darchei Chayim* helped you reconnect with your inner Divine spark and use remembered strengths, resources, and coping tools in difficult circumstances. Whether your inspiration is from within, from other people, from God, from nature, or other pathways, the hope is that you will feel comforted, shepherded, and inspired. Even when the future still looks challenging, turning to spiritual resources for coping can be a gift as you co-exist with your illness.

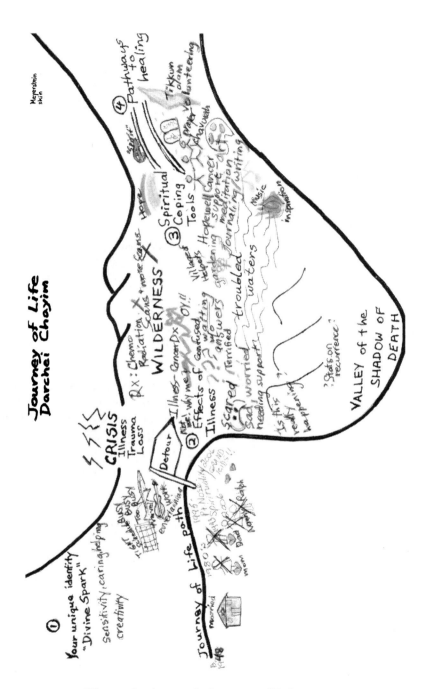

The author's sample Journey of Life map.

Chapter Fifteen

Creating Your Spiritual Treatment Plan

After doing the personal spiritual assessment and the Journey of Life exercise, now is an opportunity to create your own spiritual treatment plan. A personal spiritual treatment plan is individualized because it is for and about you. It seems only reasonable that you should create your own plan. After all, who knows you better and who should be most invested in your well-being? Jewish tradition reminds us that we have an obligation to responsibly care for our bodies and spirits. While a spiritual treatment plan can be developed in collaboration with a professional during spiritual counseling, it is also possible for you to do it on your own.

What might a Spiritual Treatment Plan include? Understand that a spiritual treatment plan is different from, but can complement, a medical treatment plan. While both are preceded by a form of assessment, a spiritual treatment plan differs both in language and spirit. It evolves out of your personal spiritual self-assessment, which should be a sincere self-reflection about your emotions and needs that will lead to some insights and a willingness to modify unhelpful habits. In short, it should reflect your potential growth through seeking constructive new pathways.

Fortunately, a wide repertoire of Spiritual Coping Tools is available to you. You can select from the practical spiritual toolbox, the treasure chest of traditional and modern coping tools, and the Biblical symbols in the Journey of Life exercise. These resources are only a starting point for you to create your own meaningful pathways of expression. Some people are naturally drawn to verbal linguistic tools, some to auditory or nonverbal pathways, and others to active doing and touching. Through their active use, these tools can strengthen a sense of coping and connection. Those who, understandably, feel too tired and burnt out right now due to illness, may need to just rest and be open to receiving support.

A Spiritual Treatment Plan can benefit us and improve our resilience in coping if we view stressful challenges as learning opportunities, and can find positive meaning in difficult situations. Orloff recommends focusing on practicing gratitude and focusing on future hopes and goals.[1] Some measure of stress may be good, if it activates us to seek better health practices (e.g. diet, nutrition, and exercise), spiritual outlets (e.g. yoga, meditation, and prayer), or motivates us to seek connection and support. "Paying it forward," by doing good deeds for others can renew our spirits as well. Perhaps a checkbook metaphor can help illustrate a point.[2] Stressors that affirm and strengthen us add credit to our account. Bad stress, or things that sap energy, debit our account. Remember, you are the banker in charge.

Another metaphor, of Jacob wrestling with angels on the ladder, can remind us of striving for goals and transformation. Climbing a ladder, even a short one, can be a daunting task requiring strength and courage. At the outset, we don't know how far up we will get. Perhaps we will feel supported if someone holds the metaphorical ladder and "spots us" as we climb. Reflecting on our strengths and receiving support may give us encouragement along the way. The climbing metaphor is echoed in the words of Rev. Martin Luther King:

> *"Take the first step in faith. You don't have to see the whole staircase, just take the first step."*

I have compiled a list of Spiritual Coping Tools from various traditions to help you create your Spiritual Treatment Plan. Which tools do you think will increase your personal agency? Help you feel less alone? More balanced and self-regulated? In the Journey of Life exercise, which symbols for strengthening did you select for comfort and inspiration? These ideas, together with your self-knowledge and creative imagination will help you create your own spiritual treatment plan.

> *"A person who saves one life, it is as if that person saved an entire world."*
>
> Talmud Sanhedrin, Ch. 4

Spiritual Coping Tools

Acupuncture
Affirmations
Ancestral wisdom
Art
Ayurveda
Bibliotherapy
Biblical symbols
Bikur Cholim
Biofeedback
Breathing
Community blessings and practices
Complementary and Alternative approaches
Diet
Exercise
Gardening
Humor
Homeopathy
Inspirational quotes
Journaling
Journey of Life (Darchei Chayim)
Mantras
Massage
Meditation (Bible, Talmud, Rabbinic)
Mindfulness
Mosaics
Music
Nature
Niggun
Nutrition
Poetry
Prayer
Psalms
Reflexology
Reiki
Rolfing
Shabbat
Songs
Stories (Hasidic, modern)
Support groups
Tai Chi
Texts
Tikkun Olam
Touch
Tzedakah
Visualization
Yoga

Caring for our bodies and souls shows responsibility and concern for our impact on others around us. Both *tikkun nefesh* and *tikkun olam* are a way of bringing further holiness into the world. In the long run, the life you save may be your own.

A World Of Responsibility

Architect of the world,
Author of her story,
Grant me the courage
To participate
In the world's design,
To join in the unfolding of her story,
How I want to share
In the responsibility of this world,
To pray for her welfare,
To care for her needs,
To work for her rectification.

Reb Nachman of Breslov

Create Your Spiritual Treatment Plan

For comfort I will seek _____

For protection I will seek _____

For strengthening I will seek _____

For learning and growth I will seek _____

For agency I will seek _____

For connection and support I will seek _____

For giving back to the community I will seek _____

Chapter Sixteen
Jewish Spiritual Coping Tool Exercises

Illness can make us forget that we have richer resources than we realize. The following chapter will provide opportunities to apply specific Jewish spiritual coping tools to help with calming anxiety, dealing with impasses, and finding meaning.

An Attitude Of Gratitude

A humble attitude of expressing gratitude regularly for life's blessings can lift our spirits. In Judaism, gratitude permeates the many daily prayers concerned with bodily health. My daily *"dovening"* (praying) trilogy consists of three prayers of gratitude: *Modeh Ani/ Asher Yatzar/ Elohai Neshama.* I sing them to contemporary melodies while walking in nature, an activity which itself evokes feelings of awe about life.

The daily practice of saying the following prayer, like a mantra, the first moment we are awake, strengthens our awareness of the great blessing of being alive.

> *Modeh Ani Lefanecha, Melech Chai V'kayam. Sheh-he-chehzarta bee nishmatee b'chemla rabbah emunatecha – I am grateful to You, living and enduring King, for returning my soul to me with compassion. Great is Your trustworthiness.*
>
> Morning Liturgy, Siddur

As you start your day, what are some of the blessings for which you are grateful? What feelings of gratitude to God can you express for the gift of life, or to others, for sustaining you? At the end of each day, try to focus on some aspect of your day, yourself, or family members for which you are grateful.

Asher Yatzar – The Gift Of My Body

Praised are You, Adonai our God, Sovereign of the Universe, Who with wisdom fashioned the human body, and Who created many orifices and many pathways. It is known and revealed that if even one of them fails, by either being blocked or opened, it would be impossible to function and to stand before Your throne of honor.

Praised are You, Adonai, Healer of all flesh, Who has made us wondrously.

The human body is made up of intricate passageways that must open or close for optimal functioning. Reading the *Asher Yatzar* prayer in English and/or Hebrew may help you reflect on the miraculous design of our bodies that enables them to work automatically ... at least most of the time. Saying the prayer expresses gratitude for smooth functioning.

I apply this prayer whenever I go for blood work. As I sit in the technician's chair I close my eyes, focus on my breathing, and use my imagination to visualize my blood flowing wondrously through my veins. This is helpful as I soon become more relaxed, and it even seems to increase the technician's success at finding a vein.

Try this. As you breathe, just notice areas of comfort and discomfort in your body. Perhaps you may want to express a prayer for continued or renewed functioning of some part of your body or your whole body.

Consider too, that open and closed tubes can refer to more than just the physical aspect of our bodies. Imagine them referring symbolically to channels of communication and relationships between people. Are there areas of relationship or communication with others that you wish would function better either by opening or closing? Could saying *Asher Yatzar* take on additional meaning in expressing these prayerful aspirations?

Elohai Neshama – The Gift Of My Soul / Spirit

The following prayer focuses on our breath and the Divine spark in each of us. The act of physical breathing reminds us of the spiritual concept of *"tzelem elokim"* and encourages us to emulate the Divine as we relate to other people and the world.

> *Elohai neshama shenatata bee tehora hee. Atah beratah, atah yetzarta, atah nefakhta bee, v'atah meshamrah bekeerbee.* – *My God, the soul which You have given me is pure. You created it, You formed it, You breathed it into me. You keep body and soul together.*
>
> Morning Liturgy, Siddur

I often recite this prayer when I go out walking. I imagine the air coming into my lungs with God's breath giving me strength and inspiration to move. As you read the prayer in Hebrew and/or English, try to reflect on your Divine breath. As you concentrate on breathing in and out naturally, notice how peaceful breathing can make you feel. Imagine a Higher Power breathing life and spirit into you, with each breath reminding you of your Divine nature.

How does having a personal sense of Divine breath inside you make you feel?

Constructing Personal Prayers

Personal prayers have long been part of man's relationship to a Higher Power, modeled after Moses' prayer in the Bible on behalf of his ill sister Miriam (Numbers 11). The prayer *"El na refa na la"* is a personal plea to heal someone. You can recite or chant the prayer, keeping in mind a person, female or male, who is in need of healing, or even say it for yourself. For a woman, the phrase ends with "La;" for a man, "Lo;" and "Li" for yourself.

In writing a personal prayer on behalf of someone, the traditional form is to address God: *Yehi Ratzon Milfanecha – May it be Your Will O God* ... and then insert your request. You might address a quality or characteristic of God that can help you. For example: "May it be Your Will, O God, Architect of the World,

Please help me plan and structure my life wisely." Another form would be: *Achat Sha'altee – One thing I ask for...* and state what you need or want followed by "Please help me to achieve it."

You can also copy a prayer onto a small prayer card and keep it at your bedside in the hospital, or give it to a friend in need. Whether you select an original or borrowed prayer, what matters is that it comes from the heart. Try constructing an original prayer and then write it on a card to carry with you.

Coping With Anxiety, Impasses, And Challenges

Anxiety is a widespread condition, reflecting our sense of true vulnerability in the world. You might find that jotting down a list of some of your fears helps recognize and contain them. The journaling I did before my emergency hysterectomy helped me manage my fears and prepare me for the upcoming surgery and all that it represented.

I remember a time when I was about to undergo foot surgery. As I lay on the operating table, panic began to set when I heard the buzzing of the surgeon's saw and realized that my anesthesia hadn't yet taken effect. I scrambled to use my imagination to create a visualization of lying on a beautiful green field of grass on a sunny day. Using my imagination, I turned the buzzing saw into a helicopter with a loud buzzing noise appearing overhead in the sky. Focusing on the beautiful day and the remote noise coming from the "helicopter" above helped me cope just long enough until the anesthesia took over.

You may want to do some regular breathing and observe where the fear seems to reside in your body. Continue to breathe in and out, saying "breathing in" and "breathing out." Imagine breathing in God's protecting love alongside the fear, and then gently releasing the fear and tension with the out breath. Alternatively, you may want to select or create your own visualization that gives you a sense of comfort and peace.

Dealing With Impasses: A Psalm For Calm

Psalms have traditionally comforted people in distress. Psalm 118 that follows refers to a situation of narrowness and feeling

Min hamaytzar karati yah, ana-nee ba-merchav-ya.

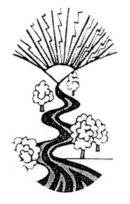

Out of the
narrow place,
I call to You, God.

Answer me with
Your expansiveness.

Psalm 118

stuck, such as when a person is ill or facing overwhelming difficulties. The antidote for this narrow state is to seek expanded options, recover prior strengths, and find solutions that free up a person to respond more flexibly.

I have used this Psalm to help myself in such situations. Reciting or singing the Psalm clip to myself creates a vital pause that allows my cognitive brain to become engaged and help me plan a more flexible response. I have also shared it numerous times with patients who are feeling stuck in interpersonal situations and don't know how to respond to an overpowering family member or friend. In a way, Psalm 118 epitomizes a therapeutic healing process, going from paralysis to constructive action.

As you look at the illustration, try to think of a situation of narrowness you have had or are experiencing. How does it make you feel? What are you struggling with? My colleague, Rabbi Gila Ruskin, would ask: "What is your *maytzar* or narrow place about?" You can use symbols, descriptive words, (sounds, smells, emotions), and colors to illustrate your experience.

What strengths can you remember calling upon that helped

you handle past situations with seemingly narrowed options or clouded perspective? What inspiration did you draw on then to cope and overcome the impasse? Which could be applied to the current situation? Recite the Psalm for calming and seeking inspiration to help you find solutions and wider options.

What helped you widen your perspective? (*merchav*). Reflecting back, what are some additional unexplored options for the situation?

Psalm Clips

Read the list of Psalm clips and select one that resonates with you. Think about how you might use it personally or on a *Bikur Cholim* visit. You may want to write it on a piece of paper and keep it with you in your wallet or pocket. Then you can take it out whenever you need inspiration to cope.

"God is near to those that are of a broken heart."

Psalm 34:19

"I lift my eyes up to the mountains from where my help will come."

Psalm 121:1

"They that sow in tears shall reap in joy."

Psalm 126:5

"Yea, though I walk through the valley of the shadow of death, I will fear no evil for You are with me."

Psalm 23:4

"Do not cast me away when I am old; do not forsake me when my strength is gone."

Psalm 71:9

"Teach us to number our days that we may get a heart of wisdom."

Psalm 90:1

Inspiring Words

Alternatively, you may want to write your own words of inspiration to carry with you, such as "hope," "perseverance," "courage," "love," on slips of paper or smooth rocks. Reciting positive affirmations about yourself and recording good deeds and qualities you possess can help convince you of the truth that **God absolutely doesn't make junk!**

Pick an inspiring quote or even a one-word anthem such as: "Believe," "Inspiration," or "Recovery" to post on a wall or keep with you to look at frequently.

Becoming A Blessing

Think about some of the ways you bring light into the world. What *mitzvot* (good deeds) do you perform? How can you continue to be a blessing to yourself and others?

You might want to light a candle, take a moment to observe its glow, and then read the following inspirational blessing for yourself.

> *May I be patient and present in all that I do.*
> *May I practice "hakarat hatov" and recognize the good in others.*
> *May I be inspired to help repair the world.*
> *May I open my heart with compassion and be a healing presence for others.*
> *May I find ways to renew my spirit when weary.*
> *May I care for myself and always find my strengths.*
> Israela Meyerstein

In the future, what are some ways I can bring light and contribute to increase holiness in the world?

Postscript

Thank you for taking this journey with me. I hope you have found expanded pathways for coping with illness and other challenges. While going through your present travails, I believe you'll find that developing a forward focus and making plans for future milestones creates a more hopeful orientation. The word "*Chaim*" in Biblical Hebrew refers to "life" and "recovery." Wherever we are in life, we can aim to improve and grow.

I like Emerson's views on attaining the age of mastery.

Definition Of A Successful Life

To laugh often and much;
to win the respect of intelligent people
and the affection of children;
to earn the appreciation of honest critics
and endure the betrayal of false friends;
to appreciate beauty, to find the best in others;
to leave the world a bit better;
whether by a healthy child,
a garden patch or a redeemed social condition;
to know even one life has breathed easier
because you have lived.

Ralph Waldo Emerson

My encounter with illness and subsequent journey through treatment and recovery heightened my awareness of our transient nature on earth and the mystery of life. None of us knows how much time we have. However, it is not just about length of our days, but how we fill them. That makes our time very precious. Illness and injury beckon us to carefully decide how to spend our limited quantity of time in a quality way. Each of us must develop a satisfying balance of focusing on obligations to self, family, community, and the larger world. It is a task that constitutes the art of life and may take a lifetime. I recently found a lovely quote that resonates with me at this point in my life:

"Don't ask what the world needs. Ask what makes you come alive and go do it. Because what the world needs are people who have come alive."

Howard Thurman
Theologian, educator, and civil rights leader

My hope is that reading this book will encourage you to use a practical spiritual perspective to better understand your song or task in the universe. Finding purpose in life is an ongoing task since meaning is not just discovered; it must be constructed. Building a repertoire of down-to-earth spiritual coping tools to strengthen ourselves from within is a tremendously valuable investment in health and well-being.

As we continue our journeys in life, may we all use ourselves fully to seek personal health and well-being, and contribute to the repair of the world so as to merit the blessings that we have been given.

PART V
NOTES AND REFERENCES

Endnotes

Note

1 The dating format in this book is Month/Day/Year.

2 For all supporting material included in this book, the author has received permission from the copyright holders and/or followed the doctrine of "Fair Use" within copyright law. The author has diligently attributed her sources for supporting material referenced in this book.

❦

1 *Stems Out Of Scratches*: Adapted by Simkha Y. Weintraub from Heinemann B. (1978) *The Maggid of Dubno and His Parables*. Heinemann, New York: Feldheim Publishers, 142-143.

Introduction

1 American Cancer Society, (2013), Cancer Facts & Figures. Retrieved from http://www.cancer.org/acs/groups/content@ epidemiologysurveillance/documents/document/acspc-036845.pdf

2 Jackson Nakazawa, D. (2009), Ill in a day's work. More Magazine, February 2009, 129-135.

3 Institute of Medicine of the National Academies, (2013), Returning home from Iraq and Afghanistan; Assessment of readjustment needs of veterans, service members, and their families. Report Brief, March 2013, The National Academy of Sciences, 1

4 Margolis, S. (Ed.) Avoiding caregiver burnout. Johns Hopkins Medicine, Health after 50. Vol. 25:14, Winter, 2013-14. (JHHealthAlerts.com)

5 Griffith, J. L. (2010), Religion That Heals, Religion that Harms: A Guide for Clinical Practice. New York: Guilford Press.

Chapter One

1 Heschel, A. J. (1964), The Patient as a Person, Conservative Judaism, Vol. XIX No.1, Fall 1964. New York: The Rabbinical Assembly, 1-10.

2   Cummings, N. (2009), Finding new clients in health care. In Cooper, Clinicians' Digest, *Psychotherapy Networker,* Jan/Feb. 2009, 18.

3   Barsky, A. J. (1981), Hidden reasons some patients visit doctors. *Annals of Internal Medicine,* 94:492-98.

4   Arden, J. & Linford, L. (2010), The rise and fall of Pax Medica. *Psychotherapy Networker,* Jan/Feb 2010.

5   Lipton, B. (2005), *The Biology of Belief: Unleashing the Power of Consciousness, Matter, and Miracles.* Mountains of Love.

6   Pargament, K.I. (1997), *The Psychology of Religion and Coping: Theory, Research, and Practice.* New York: Guilford.

7   Brody, H. (2000), *The Placebo Response: How You Can Release the Body's Inner Pharmacy for Better Health.* New York: Harper Collins.

8   Green, A. (2012), Restoring the Aleph: Judaism for the Contemporary Seeker. *Institute for Jewish Spirituality.*

9   Bateson, G. & Bateson, M.C. (1987), *Angels Fear: Towards an Epistemology of the Sacred,* New York: Macmillan.

10   Thoresen, C.E. (1998), Spirituality, health, and science: The coming revival? In S. Roth-Roemer, S. Kurplus, & C. Carmin (Eds.), *The Emerging Role of Counseling Psychology in Health Care.* New York: Norton, 409-431.

11   Wicker, C. (2009), How spiritual are we? *Parade Magazine* (10/4/09). A recent study found that 69% of Americans believe in God, 77% pray outside religious services, 24% consider themselves "spiritual but not religious," and 27% don't practice. 51% pray daily, of which 72% pray for others, 60% pray for forgiveness, 27% for personal success, and 21% for money and material things.

12   Rosenberg, J. (1993), Faith in medicine. *American Medical News,* 12/20/93, 15-18.

13   Butler, K. (1990), Psychotherapy and Spirituality: Rethinking age old questions. *Psychotherapy Networker,* 5, 279-287.

14   Helmeke, K. B., Bischoff, G.H. (2002), Recognizing and raising spiritual and religious issues in therapy: Guidelines for the timid. *Journal of Family Psychotherapy, 13,1/2,* 195-214.

15   Frame, M. W. (2000), The spiritual genogram in family therapy. *Journal of Marital and Family Therapy,* 26: 211-216.

16 Hodge, D. R. (2000), Spiritual Ecomaps: A new diagrammatic tool for assessing marital and family spirituality, *Journal of Marital and Family Therapy,* 2, 217-28.

17 Carlson, T. D., Kirkpatrick, D., Hecker, L., & Kellner, M, (2002), Religion, spirituality, and marriage and family therapy: A study of family therapists; beliefs about the appropriateness of addressing spiritual issues in therapy. *American Journal of Family Therapy,* 30, 157-171.

18 Larson, D. B. (2001), Spirituality-the forgotten factor in health and mental health; what does the research say? *Institute for Professional Development,* Jewish Family Services, Baltimore, MD, 1/18/01.

19 Levin, J. (2001), *God, Faith and Health: Exploring the Spirituality-Healing Connection.* New York: Wiley.

20 Kaslow, F. & Robinson, J. A. (1996), Long-term satisfying marriages: perceptions of contributing factors. *American Journal of Family Therapy,* 24 (2), 153-170.

21 Benson, H. & Stark, M. (1996), *Timeless Healing: The Power and Biology of Belief.* New York: Fireside.

22 Dossey, L. (1993), *Healing Words: The Power of Prayer and the Practice of Medicine.* San Francisco: Harper.

23 Matthews, D. A. (1998), *The Faith Factor: Proof of the Healing Power of Prayer.* New York: Viking Penguin.

24 Walsh, F. (1998), Transcendence. In M. McGoldrick (Ed.), *Re-visioning Family Therapy: Race, Culture, and Gender in Clinical Practice.* New York: Guilford, 62-77.

25 Griffith, J. L. & Griffith, M. E. (2001), *Encountering the Sacred in Psychotherapy: How to Talk with People about their Spiritual Lives.* New York: Guilford.

26 Hirschberg, C. & Barasch, M. I, (1995), *Remarkable Recovery: What Extraordinary Healings Tell Us About Getting Well and Staying Well.* New York: Riverhead.

27 Seddon, C. (2009), Personal communication. 9/27/09.

28 Lamm, M. (1995), *The Power of Hope: The One Essential of Life and Love.* New York: Fireside Books.

29 Antoni, M. H. & Carver, C.S. (2003), Cognitive behavioral stress management interventions and positive psychological changes in

breast cancer patients after surgery and their physiological correlates. *Proceedings of the American Society of Clinical Oncology*, 22, Abstract No. 3064, 762.

30   Helgeson, V., Cohen, S., Schulz, R., Yasko, I. (1999), Education and peer discussion group interventions and adjustment to breast cancer. *Archives of General Psychiatry*, 56, 340-347.

31   Gonzalez, S., Steinglass, P., & Reiss, D. (1989), Putting the illness in its place: Discussion groups for families with chronic medical illness. *Family Process*, 28:69-87.

32   Steinglass, P. (1998), Multiple family discussion groups for patients with chronic medical illness. *Families, Systems, and Health*, Vol. 16, Nos. 1/2, 55-70.

33   Cooper, G. (2003), Clinical Update, *Psychotherapy Networker.* May/June, 13-14.

34   Moran, M. (2002), Cancer group Therapy adds to well-being, not longevity. *Professional News*, Jan. 18, 2002.

35   Meyerstein, I. (2005), Sustaining Our Spirits: Spiritual Study/Discussion Groups for Coping with Medical Illness. *Journal of Religion and Health*, 44, No. 2, 207-226.

36   The anecdote, the origin of which is not known, was included in Rabbi Harold Kushner's book, *When All You've Ever Wanted Isn't Enough: The Search for a Life that Matters.* Rabbi Kushner is happy to have us share it. (Personal communication, 7/13/14).

37   Butler, K. (1990), Spirituality reconsidered: Facing the limits of psychotherapy. In Psychotherapy and Spirituality: Rethinking Age-Old Questions. *The Family Therapy Networker,* Sept /Oct. 1990, 26-37, 30.

38   Simonton, C. O., cited in Oz, M. C. with R. Arias & L. Oz (1999), *Healing from the Heart: A Leading Surgeon Reveals How Unconventional Wisdom Unleashes the Power of Modern Medicine,* New York: Plume.

39   Greenspan, M. (2003), Healing Through the Dark Emotions: The Wisdom of Grief, Fear, and Despair. Boston: Shambala Publications.

40   Remen, R. N. (1992), Final Endings, *Beyond cure: Four talks on healing for health professionals.* Bolinas, CA: Institute for the Study of Health and Illness.

41   Remen, R.N. (2000), Reclaiming the Heart and Soul of the Health Professional. *Washington Hospital Center Workshop.* Washington, DC, 6/19/00.

Chapter Two

1   Jonathan Omer Man, cited as personal communication in N. Flam (2001), Spiritual Nurture for Jewish Pastoral Caregivers. In D.A. Friedman (Ed.), *Jewish Pastoral Care: A Practical Handbook.* From Traditional and Contemporary Sources. Woodstock, VT: Jewish Lights Publishing.

2   Tanakh, (1985), The Holy Scriptures. The New JPS Translation According to the Traditional Hebrew Text. Philadelphia, PA: The Jewish Publication Society, Genesis 18:1.

3   Ibid, Numbers 12:13.

4   Ibid, Kings II Chapter 4, v. 32-34.

5   Epstein, I. (Ed.) (1936), The Babylonian Talmud, Eight Volumes, London: Soncino Press, Berakhot 5b.

6   Ibid, Nedarim 39b.

7   Meyerstein, I. & Ruskin, G. (2007), Spiritual tools for enhancing the pastoral visit to hospitalized patients. *Journal of Religion and Health,* 46, 1, 109-122.

8   Green, A. (1992), *Tormented Master: The Life and Spiritual Quest of Rabbi Nahman of Bratslav.* Woodstock, VT: Jewish Lights Publishing.

9   Likutey Moharan 1:29, 1-2.

10   Buettner, D. (2008), Find purpose, live longer, add years to your life by adding life to your years, *AARP,* Nov.-Dec. 2008, 32.

Note: Research shows that people with purpose have a stronger immune system, lower risk of heart attack and cancer, heal faster, and live longer. Buettner, D. (2008), *The Blue Zone: Lessons for Living Longer from the People who've lived the Longest,* National Geographic.

Chapter Three

1   Herbert, W. (2006), The passing of a visionary. *Psychotherapy Networker,* Sept. / Oct., 2006, 30:5, 17-18.

2 Helgeson, V. S. (1993), Implications of agency and communion for patient and spouse adjustment to a first coronary event. *Journal of Personality and Social Psychology, 64:5*, 807-816.

3 Helgeson, V. S. (1992), Moderators of the relation between perceived control and adjustment to chronic illness. Journal of Personality and Social Psychology, 63:4, 656-666.

4 Berkman, L. F. & Syme, L. (1979), Social networks, host resistance, and mortality: A nine-year follow-up study of Alameda County residents. *American Journal of Epidemiology,* 109:2. 186-204.

5 Cohen, S. (1990), Social support and physical illness. *Advances, Institute for the Advancement of Health,* 7:1, 35-48.

6 Sagan, L. A. (1990), The social networks of health. Advances: Institute for the Advancement of Health, 4. 5-17.

7 McGonigal, K.(2013), "How to make stress your friend." Ted Global, Edinburgh, Scotland, 6/13.

Chapter Four

1 Weintraub, S.Y. (2007), Mi Sheberach for Health Care Professionals. In Marcus, J. & Dickstein, S. (Editors), Jewish Spiritual Companion for Medical Treatments, National Center for Jewish Healing & Twin Cities Jewish Healing Program, 21.

2 Maimonides, *Matanot Ani'im* (Laws of Gifts to Poor People).

Chapter Five

1 Silver, M. (2004), *Breast Cancer Husband: How to Help Your Wife (And Yourself) Through Diagnosis, Treatment, and Beyond.* Rodale Press.

2 Ibid.

3. Heschel, A. J. (1964), The patient as a person. Conservative Judaism: Vol XIX, Number 1, Fall 1964. New York: The Rabbinical Assembly.

4 Neely, S. K., McInorff, W. D. & Cohen, J. J. (1998), What Americans Say About the Nations' Medical Schools and Teaching Hospitals, *Report on Public Opinion Research, Part II.* Washington, D.C.: Association of American Medical Colleges, 9.

5 Oglesby, P. (1991), *The Caring Physician: The Life of Dr. Francis W.*

Peabody. Cambridge, MA: Harvard University Press.

6   Siegel, D. (1980), *Angels.* Town House, Inc. p.52A.

7   Burnham, S. (1990), *A Book of Angels; Reflections on Angels Past and Present, and True Stories of How They Touch Our Lives.* New York: Ballantine Books.

8   Friedman, D. (1995), Al Tasteir, Renewal of Spirit, San Diego, CA: Sounds Write Productions.

Chapter Six

1   Singer, Simeon, (1915), The Standard Prayer Book.

2   Friedman, D. (1995), *Renewal of Spirit.* Sounds Write Productions, Inc.

3   Naparstek, B. (1991), *A Meditation to Help You with Chemotherapy.* Healthjourneys. (www.healthjourneys.com)

Chapter Seven

No endnotes for this chapter.

Chapter Eight

1   Newman, J. (2010), Living after cancer. *Parade Magazine* 6/20/10. P.5. Note: There are well over twelve million survivors in the United States alone, a number that has tripled in thirty years, of whom 25% had multiple cancers, and 18 million survivors are predicted by 2022. American Cancer Society (2013) estimates 13.7 million survivors today.

2   Rosen, J. (2009), What else survivors face: New awareness of after effects leads to long-term support, *The Baltimore Sun,* 10/26/09.

3   Zampini, K. & Ostroff, J. S. (1993), The post- treatment resource program: Portrait of a program for cancer survivors. *Psycho-Oncology, 2,* 1-9.

4   Frellick, M. (2009), Living as a breast cancer survivor. *Health section, The Baltimore Sun,* 10/26/09, p.12. Note: Forty percent of American cancer survivors are of working age.

5   Ibid.

6   Siegel-Itzkowich, J., (2012), How to bring the loving back after cancer, *The Jerusalem Post,* 3/14/12, 1-4.

7   Pash, B. (2013), Mistletoe's the mission for cancer survivor. The Baltimore Sun, News, (9/22/13), 10.

8   Carmichael, M. (2009), Who says stress is bad for you? *Newsweek,* 2/19/09, p. 1-5. www.newsweek.com/id/184154/output/print..

9   Kaiser Stearns, A. (2010), *Living Through Personal Crisis; A Compassionate Guide for Triumphantly Surviving Difficult Events and For Helping Loved Ones and Friends.* Enumclaw, WA: Idyll Arbor, Inc.

Chapter Nine

1   Kushner, H. S. (2004), *When Bad Things Happen to Good People.* New York: Anchor Books.

2   American Cancer Society (2006), *Listen with Your Heart: Talking with the Person who has Cancer.*

3   Patterson, J. M. & Garwick, A. W. (1994), Levels of meaning in family stress theory. *Family Process,* 33 (3), 287-304.

4   Antonovsky, A. (1979), *Health, Stress, and Coping.* San Francisco: Jossey Bass Publishers.

5   D'Adamo, P. J., with Catherine Whitney, (2001), *Live Right for Your Type: The Individualized Prescription for Maximizing Health, Metabolism, and Vitality in Every Stage of Your Life.* New York: C. P. Putnam's Sons.

6   Ibid.

7   Servan-Schreiber, D. (2009), The anti-cancer lifestyle: A promising new strategy for avoiding a killer disease-or keeping it from coming back, *Health Report. AARP,* March/April 2009, 24, 26-27.

8   Gupta, S. (2007), *Chasing Life: New Discoveries in the Search for Immortality to Help You Age Less today.* New York: Warner Wellness.

9   Servan-Schreiber, D. (2009), The anti-cancer lifestyle: A promising new strategy for avoiding a killer disease – or keeping it from coming back, *Health Report. AARP,* March/April 2009, 24, 26-27.

10   Wolfe, D. L. (2006), *Reclaim Your Inner Terrain,* Fourth Edition, The Wolfe Clinic.

11   Cook, M. S. (2008), *The Ultimate pH Solution: Balance Your Body Chemistry to Prevent Disease and Lose Weight.* New York: Harper Collins.

12   Cabot, R. C. (1909), *Social Service and the Art of Healing.* New York: Moffat, Yard, & Co.

13   Nee, L.E. (1995), Effects of psychosocial interaction at a cellular level. *Social Work,* 40/2, March 1995, 259-262.

14   Carmichael, M. (2009), Why Stress May be Good for You. *Newsweek,* 2/13/09.

15   Ader, R., Felton, D. & Cohen, N. (1990), Interaction between the brain and the immune system. *Annual Review of Pharmacological Toxicology,* 30, 561-2.

16   Weihs, K. L., Enright, T.M., Simmons, S. J., Reiss, D. (2000), Negative affectivity, restriction of emotions, and site of metasteses predict mortality in recurrent breast cancer. Journal of Psychosomatic Research 49 (1), 59-68.

17   Greenspan, M. (2004), *Healing Through the Dark Emotions: The Wisdom of Grief, Fear, and Despair.* Shambala.

18   Friedman, E. H. (1985), Body and Soul in Family Process. In *Generation to Generation: Family Process in Church and Synagogue.* New York: Guilford Press, 121-146.

19   Friedman, E. H. (1986), Resources for healing and survival in families. In M.A. Karpel, *Family Resources: The Hidden Partner in Family Therapy.* New York: The Guilford Press, 65-92.

20   Meyerstein, I. (1994), Reflections on "being there" and "doing" in family therapy: A story of chronic illness, *Family Systems Medicine,* 12:1, 21-29.

21   Hinderberger, P. (1995), Personal communication. 9/14/95.

Chapter Ten

1   Meyerstein, I. (1994), Reflections on "being there" and "doing" in family therapy: a story of chronic illness, *Family Systems Medicine,* 10:1, 99-110.

2   Pauch, R. with Zaslow, J, (2008), *The Last Lecture.* New York: Hyperion.

3   Williamson, M. (1992), *A Return to Love; Reflections on the Principles of a Course in Miracles.* New York: Harper Collins.

4   Lamm, M. (1995), *The Power of Hope; The One Essential of Life and Love.* New York: Fireside. (1997).

Chapter Eleven

1   Caldwell, K. (2010), Is it conventional, complementary, alternative, or integrative? (medicine, that is). *Family Therapy Magazine: Alternative Therapies,* March/ April 2010, 23.

2   Nakin, R. L., Barnea, P.M., Stussman, B. J., Bloom, B. (2009), *Costs of complementary and alternative medicine and frequency of visit to CAM practitioners.* United States 2007 National Health Statistics Report. No. 18. Hyattsville, Md.; National Center for Health Statistics.

3   Jaret, P. (2010), *Battling Cancer.* http://bulletin.aarp.org, 10-12.

4   Izzo, A. A. & Ernst, E. (2001), *Interactions between herbal medicines and prescribed drugs: a systemic review, Drugs,* 61(15), 2163-2175

5   Caldwell, K. (2010), Is it conventional, complementary, alternative, or integrative? (medicine, that is). *Family Therapy Magazine: Alternative therapies.* March/ April 2010.

6   NCCAM (2010), Acupuncture and Pain: Applying modern science to an ancient practice. *Complementary and Alternative Medicine: Focus on Research and Care,* National Institute of Health, Feb. 2010, 3.

7   Ibid.

8   Oz, M. C. with R. Arias & L. Oz (1998), *Healing From the Heart.* New York: Plume.

9   Personal communication. Maureen O'Brien. Chaplain, St. Joseph Hospital, Baltimore, MD.

10   Ungless, J. (2010), Stretch your way out of stress. *More Magazine,* Dec/Jan, 156, 158.

11   Milgrom, J. (1994), *Handmade Midrash.* Philadelphia, Pa.: Jewish Publication Society.

12   Gesell, I. & Trieber, R, (2008), *Cancer and the Healing Power of Play: A Prescription for Living Joyously with Presence, Acceptance, and Trust.* US: Instant Publisher.

13 Khatchadourian, R. (2010), The laughing guru: Madan Kataria's prescription for total well-being. *The New Yorker,* 8/30/10, 56-60.

14 Cousins, N. (1979), *Anatomy of an Illness as Perceived by the Patient,* New York: W.W. Norton & Co.

15 Penn, P. (2001), Chronic illness: Trauma, language, and writing: breaking the silence. *Family Process,* 40:1, 33-51.

16 Pennebaker, J. W, (1993), Putting stress into words: Health, linguistics, and therapeutic Implications, *Behavior, Research, and Therapy,* 31, 539-547.

17 Sachs, O. (2002), When music heals, *Parade Magazine.* 3/31/02, 4-5.

18 Oz, M. C. with R. Arias & L. Oz, (1998), *Healing From the Heart.* New York: Plume, 98.

19 Benson, H. & Kipper, M. (1975), *The Relaxation Response.* New York: William Morrow.

20 Freeman, D.L. & Abrams, J. Z. (1999), *Illness and Health in the Jewish Tradition: Writings from the Bible to Today,* Philadelphia, Pa.: Jewish Publication Society.

21 Gaynor, M. L. (1999), *Sounds of Healing: A Physician Reveals the Therapeutic Power of Sound, Voice, and Music,* New York: Broadway Books.

22 Oz, M. C. with R. Arias & L. Oz (1998), *Healing from the Heart: A Leading Surgeon Reveals How Unconventional Wisdom Unleashes the Power of Modern Medicine.* New York: Plume.

23 Benson, H & Kipper, M. (1975), *The Relaxation Response.* New York: William Morrow.

24 Carlson, L. E. & Brown, K. W. (2005), Validation of the mindful attention Awareness scale in a cancer population. *Journal of Psychosomatic Research,* 58, 29-33.

25 Elliman, W. (1989), The patient in control. *Hadassah Magazine.* April 1989, 34-36.

26 Siegel, D. (2007), *The Mindful Brain: Reflection and Attunement in the Cultivation of Well Being.* New York: W.W. Norton.

27 Newberg, A., D'Aquilli, T., Rause, V. (2001), *Why God Won't Go Away: Brain Science and The Biology of Belief.* New York: Ballantine.

28 Bhanoo, S. N., (2011), How meditation may change the brain. http:// well.blogs.nytimes.com, 1/28/11.

29 Kornfeld, J. & Fronsdal, G. (Eds.), (1993), *Teachings of the Buddha.* Boston: Shambala.

30 Olitzky, K.M. (2000), *Jewish Paths Toward Healing and Wholeness: A Personal Guide to Dealing with Suffering,* Woodstock, Vt.: Jewish Lights Publishing.

31 *Cancer Self-Help Education,* (1977), Health Education Programs, Cancer Counseling & Research Center, Saratoga, CA.

32 *When the Body Hurts, the Soul Still Longs to Sing,* (1992), Jewish Healing Center, San Francisco, CA.

33 Friedman, D. (1995), *The Angels' Blessing. Renewal of Spirit* CD. Music by Debbie Friedman, Lyrics by Debbie Friedman and D'rora Setel. Sounds Write Productions, Inc.

34 Patton Thoele, S. (1998), *The Woman's Book of Soul: Meditations for Courage, Confidence, and Spirit.* New York: MJF Books.

35 Frank, O.M., Pressler, M. (Eds.), Massotty, S. (Transl.), (1997), *Anne Frank, The Diary of a Young Girl: The Definitive Edition,* New York: Doubleday.

36 Scherman, N. (Transl. & Insights), (2005), *Perek Shirah: The Song of the Universe.* Brooklyn, NY: Mesorah Publications, Ltd.

37 Weintraub, S. Y. (2007), A Nature Prayer, Adapted from Likutey Moharan, Part I, #52 by Reb Nachman of Breslov. In Marcus, J. & Dickstein, S. (Eds.), *Jewish Spiritual Companion for Medical Treatments,* New York: The National Center for Jewish Healing/ Jewish Board of Family and Children's Services, 14.

Chapter Twelve

1 Oz, M. with R. Arias & L. Oz. (1998), *Healing From the Heart.* USA: Plume.

2 Ibid.

3 Flam, N., Offel, J., & Eilberg, A. (1995), *Acts of Loving-kindness: A Training Manual for Bikkur Cholim.* New York: National Center for Jewish Healing.

4 Synagogue 3000, (2009), *Spirituality at Bnai Jeshurun: Reflections of Two Scholars and Three Rabbis.* Los Angeles, CA: S3K Synagogue Studies Institute.

5   Roof, W. C, (1993), *A Generation of Seekers: The Spiritual Journeys of the Baby Boomer Generation.* San Francisco, CA: Harper.

6   Shulman, R.J. (Ed.), (2013), Siddur *Hinneni* "Here I Am" Fourth Edition.

7   Wilferd Arlan Peterson, according to Wikipedia, (en.wikipedia.org/ wiki/Wilferd_Arlan_Peterson), printed in *Signs of the Times*, 4/1/60. Others attribute it to Muir Holborn, and still others claim it is a translation on an ancient Hittite prayer from Turkey.

8   Prager, K.M. (1997), For everything a blessing: A piece of my mind. *Journal of the American Medical Association.* 5/28/97, 277:20, 1589.

9   Ornstein, D, (2008), "Angels in the outhouse": New perspectives on *Birkat Asher Yatzar. Conservative Judaism*, 22-41.

10   Singer, Simeon, (1915), The Standard Prayer Book.

11   Michaels, J. (1996), Making Your Own "Healing Card," *The Outstretched Arm*, Vol. V, Issue 3, Fall 1996, p.2, New York: The National Center for Jewish Healing.

12   Levy, N. (2002), *Talking to God: Personal Prayers for Times of Joy, Sadness, Struggle, and Celebration.* New York: Alfred A. Knopf, 35.

13   Levin, J. (2001), *God, Faith, and Health: Exploring the Spirituality-Healing Connection.* New York: Wiley.

14   Olitzky, K. M, ((2000), *Jewish Paths toward Healing and Wholeness: A Personal Guide to Dealing with Suffering.* Woodstock, Vt.: Jewish Lights Publishing.

15   Pargament, K. I, (1997), *The Psychology of Religion and Coping: Theory, Research, & Practice.* New York: Guilford.

16   Roberts, J. (1988), Setting the frame: Definition, functions, and typology of rituals, In E. Imber-Black, J. Roberts, R. Whiting (Eds.) *Rituals in Families and Family Therapy.* New York: Guilford.

17   Minkove, J. F. (2009), Saved by the Bell. www. hopkinskimmelcancercenter.org/index.cfm/cID/177... 10/25/09.

18   Blanchard, T. (1994), Sacred Scars: how storytelling heals and restores. *Sh'ma: A Journal of Jewish Responsibility, 25/479*, 10/14/94, CLAL: The National Jewish Center for Learning and Leadership.

19   Talmud, Tractate Ketubot 104a

20   Twerski, A. J. (1995), *Living Each Day.* Brooklyn, NY: Mesorah Publications, p. 335.

21   Monk Kidd, S. (1992), *When the Heart Waits: Spiritual Direction for Life's Sacred Questions (Plus).* New York: Harper Collins.

22   Spiritual story, author unknown.

23   Breger, S. (2010), *How Tikkun Olam got its groove,* Moment Magazine, May/June, 24, 27.

24   Siegel, D. (1999), "Mitzvah Therapy" in *Healing: Readings and Meditations.* Pittsboro, NC: The Town House Press.

25   Parker Pope, T, (2009), In a month of giving, a healthy reward, *New York Times,* Wellness section. 11/30/09.

26   O'Hanlon, B. (2006), *Pathways to Spirituality: Connection, Wholeness, and Possibility for Therapist and Client.* New York: W.W. Norton.

27   Walker, C. (2009), *29 Gifts: How a Month of Giving Can Change Your Life.* New York: DaCapo Press.

28   Wenner Moyer, M., (2013), Three Months to Healthy, *Parade Magazine,* 10/13/13, 9-10. Note: A meta-analysis of five long term studies reported that people who volunteered were, on average, 22% less likely to die over a period of four to seven years than similar people who didn't volunteer.

29   Siegel, D. (1999), Courage, *Healing: Readings and Meditations.* Pittsboro, NC: The Town House Press, 3.

Chapter Thirteen

1   Griffith, J.L. & Griffith, M.E. (2001), *Encountering the Sacred in Psychotherapy; How to Talk with People About Their Spiritual Lives.* New York: Guilford Press.

2   Weintraub, S.Y. (2000), Descriptives of state of the spirit. Unpublished presentation to the National Association of Jewish Chaplains Conference, February 2000.

3   Weintraub, S.Y. (2007), Seven Ways of Asking, *Jewish Spiritual Companion for Medical Treatments.* A Collaborative Project of the Twin Cities Jewish Healing Program and The National Center for Jewish Healing. 51.

4   Hodge, D.R. (2006), A template for spiritual assessment: A review of the JCAHO requirements and guidelines for implementation. Social Work 51:4, Oct. 2006, 317-326.

5   Roberts, J. (2010), Heart and Soul: Experiential Exercises for Therapists and Clients, in F. Walsh (Ed.), Spiritual Resources in Family Therapy, Second Edition, New York: The Guilford Press, 359-378.

6   Taylor, Bonita E., personal communication cited in Z. Davidowitz-Farkas, (2001), Jewish spiritual assessment. In D.A. Friedman, (Ed.) *Jewish Pastoral Care: A Practical Handbook from Traditional and Contemporary Sources.* Woodstock, VT: Jewish Lights Publishing.

7   Davidowitz-Farkas, Z. (2001), Jewish spiritual assessment. In D.A. Friedman (Ed.). *Jewish Pastoral Care: A Practical Handbook from Traditional and Contemporary Sources.* Woodstock, VT: Jewish Lights Publishing, 105-124.

8   O'Hanlon, B. (2006), *Pathways to Spirituality: Connection, Wholeness, and Possibility for Therapist and Client.* New York: W.W. Norton.

Chapter Fourteen

1   Meyerstein, I. & Ruskin, G. (1997), The Journey of LIfe (Darchei Chayim) Exercise. Unpublished exercise.

2   Steinglass, P. (1998), Multiple family discussion groups for patients with chronic medical illness. *Families, Systems, and Health,* Vol. 16, Nos. 1/2, 55-70.

3   Olitzky, K. M, (2000), *Jewish Paths toward Healing and Wholeness: A Personal Guide to Dealing with Suffering.* Woodstock, VT: Jewish Lights Publishing.

Chapter Fifteen

1   Orloff, J. (2009), Emotional Freedom: Liberate Yourself from Negative Emotions and Transform Your Life. Harmony Press.

2   Wienn, P. (2009), Weathering the Storm: How to get out from under the stress cloud-for good. Natural Solutions, Nov/Dec, 69-72.

Glossary Of Spiritual Terms

Achat Sha'altee – First words of prayer "One thing I ask of You."

Adon Olam – Prayer at the end of religious services; means "Master of the world."

Angel of Death – Angel passing over Egyptian houses that slayed firstborn Egyptian sons.

Archangel Raphael – Heavenly physician in Christianity.

Asher Yatzar – "Who created;" Morning prayer of gratitude for bodily functioning recited by observant Jews upon leaving the bathroom in the morning.

Baal Shem Tov – Rabbi who founded Hasidism in the late 18ᵗʰ century.

Bikur (Bikkur) – Visit, assessment.

Bikur (Bikkur) Cholim – Visiting the sick.

Bircat Hagomel – Blessing recited in synagogue by a person who has just survived illness, accident, or crisis.

Chametz – Leavened products forbidden during Passover.

Chamsa – Middle-eastern symbol of a hand, signifying good luck and Divine protection against the evil eye.

Chasidic (Hasidic) – Comes from the word "chesed," meaning "loving-kindness." Orthodox Jews who stem from rabbinic dynasty lines or have adopted Hasidic mores and lifestyle.

Chavurah – Friendship group.

Chutzpah – Nerve, audacity, boldness.

Darchei Chayim – Paths of life, journey of life.

Elisha – Biblical prophet.

El na refa na la – "Please God, heal her, please." The first personal prayer in the Bible, uttered by Moses on behalf of his sister, Miriam, who was struck by leprosy.

Elohai Neshama – Morning prayer affirming the Divine Breath instilled in each of us by God.

Elohim – God.

Gam Zeh Ya'avor – "This too shall pass."

Gavriel – One of four angels, representing God's strength, on the left side.

Genogram – Diagram illustrating family relationships.

Haggadah – Book read during Passover holiday Seder meal.

Hakarat Hatov – Your gratitude to others for their help extended to you.

Hashem – Substitute name for God that is acceptable to pronounce.

Hashkivenu – Lay me down prayer from Evening Liturgy.

Havdalah – Ritual ending the Sabbath on Saturday evening after dark, using wine, spices, and special intertwined, multi-wick candle. Ceremony marks the separation between the holy Sabbath and the secular days of the week.

Kabbalah – Jewish Mysticism.

Kavannah – "With meaning" or "with a direction."

Kedushah, or Holiness Code – Biblical source of ethical principles (Leviticus 19).

Ketubah – Jewish wedding certificate presented to wife that states husband's obligations.

Klezmer – Jewish folk music from Eastern Europe

JCOAHO – Joint Commission on the Accreditation of Health Organizations.

Ma Nishtana – The Four Questions, recited by the youngest child at the Passover Seder.

Manna – Special food provided by God to the Israelites during their wandering in the wilderness.

Maytzar – Narrowness, narrow straights.

Mitzrayim – Hebrew word for Egypt.

Merchav – Wideness, expansiveness.

Michael – One of the four angels, representing the likeness of God, on the right side.

Midrash – Legends about the Torah.

Mikveh – Jewish ritual bath.

Mi Sheberach – Blessing praying for good health.

Mishnah – Ancient and medieval oral commentaries on laws given to Moses in the period preceding the Talmud; Rabbinic interpretation of Bible.

Mitzvah – Good deed, positive commandment. According to traditional Jewish texts, there are 613 commandments, including visiting the sick, improving the world, helping others.

Mitzvah Therapy – Deliberate practice of doing good deeds to help others and improve the world that also helps the helper.

Modeh Ani – "I am thankful" prayer, recited in the morning service.

Moxa – Heat applied to the area, before insertion of needles, during acupuncture treatment.

Neshama – Soul.

Neshima – Breath.

Niggun – Wordless melody.

Oy – Yiddish expression of woe, worry.

Perek Shira – Ancient text about each creature's song, task, or function on earth.

Rabbi Eliezer – Rabbi in Talmud who appears in *Bikur Cholim* stories.

Rabbi Judah the Prince – Talmudic scholar of the 3rd century.

Rabbi Levi Isaac of Berdichev – Hasidic leader (1740-1809).

Rabbi Yochanan – Rabbi in Talmud who appears in *Bikur Cholim* stories.

Rachamim – Quality of mercy.

Reb, Rebbe, Rav, Rabbi – Teacher, spiritual leader.

Reb Nachman of Breslov – Founder of Breslov sect of Hasidism (1772-1810).

Rechem – Hebrew word for womb.

Refaenu – "Heal us" group prayer in community.

Refuah – "Healing, cure, remedy, medicine, recovery."

Refuah shelaymah – A full recovery of body and spirit.

Rephael – One of four angels, representing healing of God, in back.

Seder – Passover ritual.

Shabbat – Sabbath; weekly Jewish holiday of rest from Friday sundown until Saturday at dark, when three stars appear in the sky. Observant Jews do not engage in work, cooking, commerce, travel, answer phones, or use electrical appliances that are not programmable.

Shehecheyanu – Hebrew blessing expressing gratitude to God for person's having reached a certain important occasion.

Shekhinah – Feminine aspect or quality of God; thought to hover over a patient's sickbed.

Shelaymut – Hebrew word for wholeness.

Shiva – Jewish week of mourning following burial of deceased.

Shofar – Ram's horn.

Siddur, siddurim – Prayer book(s).

Sukkah – Temporary booths constructed by Israelites during wandering in the wilderness. Today, Jews observing the holiday of Sukkot build booth that remains up for eight days. Meals are to be eaten in Sukkah during holiday.

Sukkat shelomecha – "Your sukkah of peace."

Talmud – Multi-volume central collection of ethical and legal discussions, tales, and insights of Rabbis, developed in Jewish academies during first to fifth centuries C.E. Consists of commentaries on the Mishnah.

Tanakh – Hebrew Bible referred to as Old Testament.

Tehillim – Psalms.

Tikkun Hanefesh – Repair of the soul.

Tikkun Klali – "General Remedy" consisting of specific healing Psalms prescribed by Reb Nachman of Breslov.

Tikkun Olam – Repair of the world.

Torah – "Teaching." Originally referring to the Five Books of Moses, including the Ten Commandments. Meaning expanded to include Jewish study and learning.

Tzedakah – Acts of charity, from the word "tzedek," or justice.

Tzelem Elokim – Image of God. We are made in the Divine image.

Uriel –One of the four angels, representing God's light, in front.

Yahrzeit candle – Lit on the eve of anniversary of close relative's death each year.

Yehi Ratzon Milfanecha – "May it be Your will, O God." Beginning of traditional prayer request.

Zohar – Collection of Jewish mystical writings by Rabbi Isaac Luria.

Reading References

Bikur Cholim

Blanchard, T. – *Joining Heaven and Earth: Maimonides and the Laws of Bikkur Cholim.*

Cottin Pogrebin, L. – *How to be a Friend to a Friend who's Sick.*

Flam, N. & Eilberg, A. – *Acts of Loving-kindness: A Training Manual for Bikkur Cholim.*

Handler, J. & Hetherington, K. with S.L. Kelman – *Give Me Your Hand: Traditional and Practical Guidance on Visiting the Sick.*

Selib Epstein, S. – *Visiting the Sick: The Mitzvah of Bikur Cholim.*

Caregiving And Aging

Berrin, S. – *A Heart of Wisdom; Making the Jewish Journey from Midlife through the Elder Years.*

Boss, P. – *Loving someone who has Dementia: How to Find Hope while Coping with Stress and Grief.*

Jacobs, B. – *The Emotional Survival Guide for Caregivers; Looking after yourself and your Family while Helping an Aging Parent.*

Kestenbaum, Y. – *Whence My Help Come: Caregiving In The Jewish Tradition.*

Michaels, J.R. & Kozberg, C. – *Flourishing in the Later Years: Jewish Pastoral Insights on Senior Residential Care.*

Matthews, B.G. & Trainin Blank, B. – *What to Do About Mama? A Guide to Caring for Aging Family Members.*

Complementary And Alternative Medicine

American Cancer Society/D. Rosenthal – *A Complete Guide to Complementary and Alternative Cancer Therapies.*

NCCAM – What is Complementary and Alternative Medicine? National Center for Complementary and Alternative Medicine.

Weisman, R. with B. Berman – *Own Your Health; Choosing the Best from Alternative and Conventional Medicine.*

Kabat-Zinn, J. – *Full Catastrophe Living: Using the Wisdom of Your Body and Mind to Face Stress, Pain, and Illness.*

Humor

Cousins, N. – *Anatomy of an Illness as Perceived by the Patient.*

Gesell, I. & Trieber, R. – *Cancer and the Healing Power of Play: a Prescription for Living Joyously with Presence, Acceptance, & Trust.*

Illness And Health

Campbell, T.C. and Campbell, T.M. II. – *The China Study: Startling Implications For Diet, Weight Loss, and Long-Term Health.*

Kleinman, A. – *The Illness Narratives: Suffering, Healing, and the Human Condition.*

Levin, J. – *God, Faith, and Health: Exploring the Spirituality-Healing Connection.*

Silver, M. – *Breast Cancer Husband: How to Help your Wife (and Yourself) through Diagnosis, Treatment, and Beyond.*

Inspirational Wisdom

Bookman, T. – *The Busy Soul: Ten Minute Spiritual Workouts Drawn from Jewish Tradition.*

Olitzky, K.M. & Forman, L. – *Sacred Intentions: Daily Inspiration to Strengthen the Spirit based in Jewish Wisdom.*

Meditative Practices

Benson, H. & Kipper, M. – *The Relaxation Response.*

Boorstein, S. – *Don't Just Do Something, Sit There: A Mindfulness Retreat.*

Gefen, N.F. – *Jewish Meditation: How to Begin Your Practice. Life Lights: Help for Wholeness and Healing.*

Healthjourneys Resources for Mind, Body, and Spirit. www.healthjourneys. com.

Kabat-Zinn, J. – *Wherever You go, There You Are: Mindfulness Meditation in Everyday Life.*

Khalsa, D.S., Stauth, C., Borysenko, J. – *Meditation as Medicine: Activate the Power of Your Natural Healing Force.*

McDonald, Kathleen. – *How to Meditate: A Practical Guide.*

Naparstek, B. – *Staying Well with Guided Imagery: How to Harness the Power of your Imagination for Health and Healing.*

Patton Thoele, S. – *The Woman's Book of Soul: Mediations for Courage, Confidence, and Spirit.*

Siegel, D. – *The Mindful Brain: Reflection and Attunement in the Cultivation of Well Being.*

Music

Gaynor, M.L. – *Sounds of Healing: A Physician Reveals the Therapeutic Power of Sound, Voice, and Music.*

Weil, A. & Arem, K. – *Self-Healing with Sounds and Music.*

Prayer

Cardin, N.B. – *Out of the Depths I Call to You: A Book of Prayers for the Married Jewish Woman.*

Chiel, A.A. & Sandrow, E.T. – *Fountain of Life.*

Dossey, L. – *Healing Words; The Power of Prayer and the Practice of Medicine;* Also – *Prayer is Good Medicine.*

Lavie, A. (Ed.) – *A Jewish Woman's Prayer Book.*

Levy, N. – *Talking to God: Personal Prayers for Times of Joy, Sadness, Struggle, and Celebration.*

Psalms

Chiel, S. & Dreher, H. – *For thou art with Me; The Healing Power of Psalms: Renewal, Hope, and Acceptance from the World's Most Beloved Verses.*

Mitchell, S. – *A Book of Psalms: Selected and Adapted from the Hebrew.*

Perlman, D. – *Flames to Heaven: New Psalms for Healing and Praise.*

Siegel, D. – *The Lord is a Whisper at Midnight; Psalms and Prayers.*

Weintraub, S.Y. – From the Depths: The use of Psalms. In D.A. Freeman (Ed.), *Jewish Pastoral Care: A Practical Handbook from Traditional and Contemporary Sources.*

Weintraub, S.Y. – *Healing of Soul, Healing of Body: Spiritual Leaders Unfold the Strength and Solace in Psalms.*

Spirituality

Chodron, P. – *When Things Fall Apart: Heart Advice for Difficult Times.*

Frankl, V. E., – *Man's Search for Meaning: An Introduction to Logotherapy.*

Griffith, J.L. – *Religion that Heals, Religion That Harms: A Guide for Clinical Practice.*

O'Hanlon, B. – *Pathways to Spirituality: Connection, Wholeness, and Possibility for Therapist and Client.*

Kay, M. – *Living Serendipitously: Keeping the Wonder Alive.*

Kushner, H. – *When Bad Things Happen to Good People.*

Lamm, M. – *The Power of Hope: The One Essential of Life and Love.*

Newberg, A., D'Aquilli, E., Rause, V. – *Why God Won't Go Away: Brain Science and the Biology of Belief.*

Spirituality And Healing

Barasch, M. I. & Siegel, B.S. – *The Healing Path: A Soul Approach to Illness.*

Benson, H. – *Timeless Healing; The Power and Biology of Belief.*

Hirschberg, C. & Barasch, M.I. – *Remarkable Recovery: What Extraordinary Healings Tell Us about Getting Well and Staying Well.*

Siegel, B. – *Love, Medicine, and Miracles: Lessons Learned about Self-Healing from a Surgeon's Experience with Exceptional Patients.*

Walsh, F. – *Essential Spirituality: Exercises from the World's Religions to Cultivate Kindness, Love, Joy, Peace, Vision, Wisdom, and Generosity.*

Spiritual Assessment

Davidowicz-Farkas, Z. – Jewish Spiritual Assessment. In D.A. Friedman, (Ed.), *Jewish Pastoral Care: A Practical Handbook from Traditional and Contemporary Sources.*

Hodge, D. R. – Spiritual Life Maps: A client-centered pictorial instrument for spiritual assessment, planning, and intervention.

Hodge, D. R. – Spiritual Ecomaps: A new diagrammatic tool for assessing marital and family spirituality.

Jewish Spirituality

Flam, N. (Ed.)– *When the Body Hurts, the Soul Still Longs to Sing.*

Frankel, E. – *Sacred Therapy: Jewish Spiritual Teaching on Emotional Healing and Inner Wholeness.*

Frankiel, T. & Greenfeld, J. – *Minding the Temple of the Soul: Balancing Body, Mind, and Spirit through Traditional Jewish Prayer, Movement, and Meditation.*

Green, A. – *Tormented Master: The Life and Spiritual Quest of Rabbi Nachman of Bratslav.*

Kahn, D.J. (Ed.) (2008). *Life, Faith, and Cancer; Jewish Journeys through Diagnosis, Treatment, and Recovery.*

Meszler, J. B. (2010). *Facing Illness, Finding God: How Judaism Can Help You and Your Caregivers Cope When Body or Spirit Fails.*

Nachman of Breslov – *The Empty Chair: Finding Hope and Joy.*

Olitzky, K.M. – *Jewish Paths toward Healing and Wholeness: A Personal Guide to Dealing with Suffering.*

Schur, T.G.– *Illness and Crisis: Coping the Jewish Way.*

Weintraub, S.Y. with Lever, A.M. – *Guide Me Along the Way: A Jewish Spiritual Companion for Surgery.*

Marcus, J. & Dickstein, S. (Eds.), – *A Jewish Spiritual Companion for Medical Treatments.* A Collaborative Project of the Twin Cities Jewish Healing Program, JFCS of Minneapolis, and the National Center for Jewish Healing, JBFCS.

Stories

Levin, M. – *The Golden Mountain: Marvellous Tales of Rabbi Israel Baal Shem Tov and of His Great-Grandson, Rabbi Nachman.*

Taylor, D. – *The Healing Power of Stories: Creating Yourself through the Stories of Your Life.*

Terminal Illness

Brown, E. – *Happier Endings: A Meditation on Life and Death.*

Nuland, S. – *How We Die: Reflections on Life's Final Chapter.*

Puchalski, O.M. – *Spirituality and end-of-life care: A time for listening and caring.*

Rosen, E. – *Families Facing Death: Family Dynamics of Terminal Illness.*

Shapiro, R.M. – *Last Breaths: A Guide to Easing Another's Dying.*

Zirkelbach, Thelma – *Stumbling Through The Dark: A Husband and Wife's Final Year of Life Together.*

Tikkun Olam

Siegel, D. – *1+1=3 and 37 Other Mitzvah Principles to Live By.*

To find any of the books listed in this section, enter the following weblink:

http://www.mazopublishers.com/search-for-books.html

Supportive Resources

Among the following organizations, a variety of services including information, referral, resources, and/or advocacy for patients in the community and online are provided.

Annie Appleseed Project (www.annieappleseedproject.org) 561-749-0084.

Believe Big (www.believebig.org) 1-888-317-5850.

CarePages (http://www.carepages.com)

CaringBridge (http://www.CaringBridge.org)

Casey Cares Foundation (www.caseycaresfoundation.org)

Share the Care. (http://www.sharethecare.org)

Isaac N. Trainin Coordinating Council of Bikur Cholim (www.jbfcs.org/Bikurcholim) 212-632-4730.

Jewish Caring Network (www.jewishcaringnetwork.org)

National Association of Jewish Chaplains (http://www.najc.org)

Patient Advocate Foundation (www.patientadvocacy.org) 800-532-5274.

The National Center for Jewish Healing, (www.jbfcs.org/NCJH) 212-632-4500.

Alternative Approaches

The Eden Alternative (www.edenalt.com)

Cancer Information about Complementary therapies (www.mskcc.org/aboutherbs.com)

National Center for Complementary and Alternative Medicine (www.nccam.nih.gov) 1-888-644-6226.

SongWriting Works TM (www.songwritingworks.org)

Caregiver Support

AARP (www.aarp.org/families/caregiving) 1-877-333-5885.

Alzheimer's Association (www.alz.org) 800-272-3900.

Caring.com (www.caring.com) 1-800-973-1540.

Caregiver Action Network (www.caregiveraction.org) 302-772-5050.

Eldercare Locator (www.eldercare.gov) 800-677-1116.

Family Caregiver Alliance (www.caregiver.org) 800-445-8106.

Lotsa Helping Hands (www.lotsahelpinghands.com)

National Alliance for Caregiving (www.caregiving.org) 301-718-8444.

National Family Caregiver Association (www.nfcacares.org) 800-896-3650.

Next Step in Care (www.nextstepincare.org)

Soaring Words, (www.soaringwords.org) 646-674-7105.

Well Spouse Association (www.wellspouse.org) 1-800-838-0879.

Cancer Resources

The American Cancer Society (www.cancer.org) 800-227-2345.

Cancer Care, Inc. (www.cancercareinc.org) 1-800-813-4673.

Cancer Treatment Center (www.cancercenter.com) 1-888-847-7403.

Casting for Recovery (www.castingforrecovery.com) 1-888-543-3500.

Hopewell Cancer Support (www.hopewellcancersupport.org) 410-832-2719.

National Cancer Institute (http://www.cancer.gov) 301-496-6641, 800-422-6237.

Memorial Sloan-Kettering Cancer Center, (www.mskcc.org) 1-800-525-2225.

National Institute of Health (www.nih.gov/health/clinicaltrials. gov) 1-800-411-1222.

The National Coalition for Cancer Survivorship (www. canceradvocacy.org) 301-650-9127, 877-NCCS-YES.

Cancer-young adults: http://myplanet.planetcancer.org (20s & 30s) 1-855-220-7777.

www.youngsurvival.org (ages 6-39) 877-972-1011.

Concrete Services

www.breastcancerfreebies.com – wigs, hats, makeup, housecleaning, transportation... 1-800-227-2345.

Cleaning for a Reason (free housecleaning once a month for four months during treatment, with physician's note) (http://www.cleaningforareason.org) 1-877-337-3348 .

Look Good Feel Better (www.lookgoodfeelbetter.org) 800-395-LOOK.

National Association of Professional Geriatric care (www.caremanager.org) 1-520-881-8008.

Little Pink Houses of Hope-vacation respite (www.littlepink.org) 1-336-213-4733.

Turning Heads Project (http://www.turning-heads.org)

Hospice And Palliative Care

National Hospice & Palliative Care Organization (www.nhpco.org) 703-837-1500.

National Hospice Foundation (www.nationalhospicefoundation.org) 1-703-516-4928.

Hospice Association of America (www.nahc.org) 1-202-546-4759.

American College of Physicians – Home Care Guide for Advanced Cancer (http://acponline.org) 1-800-523-1546 x2600.

Pain management (www.partnersagainstpain.com) 1-888-726-7535.

(Note: The telephone numbers have been provided for your convenience, but they change frequently. Check the website for the current telephone number.)

Publications

Meyerstein, I. & Ruskin, G. (2007), Spiritual tools for enhancing the pastoral visit to hospitalized patients, *Journal of Religion and Health*, 46:1, 109-122.

Meyerstein, I. (2006), Spiritual Steps for Couples Recovering from Fetal Loss. In K. Helmeke and C. Ford Sori (Eds.), The *Therapist's Notebook for Integrating Spirituality in Counseling II: Homework, Handouts, and Activities for Use in Psychotherapy.* Haworth Press, 223-230.

— — —, (2006), Using psalms as spiritual tools in coping with medical illness. In K. Helmeke and C. Ford Sori (Eds.), *The Therapist's Notebook for Integrating Spirituality in Counseling II: Homework, Handouts, and Activities for Use in Psychotherapy.* Haworth Press, 209-216.

— — —, (2005), Sustaining our spirits: Spiritual study/discussion groups for coping with medical illness. *Journal of Religion and Health*, 44:2, 207-225.

— — —, (2004), A Jewish Spiritual Perspective on Psychopathology and Psychotherapy: A Clinician's View. *Journal of Religion and Health*, 44:1, 329-341.

— — —, (2003), The Patient Nose: A Biopsychosociospiritual Story. In J. Frykman and T. Nelson (Eds.), *Making the Impossible Difficult: Tools for Getting Unstuck*, iUniverse.

— — —, (2001), A systemic approach to fetal loss following genetic testing. *Contemporary Family Therapy*, 23(4), 385-402.

— — —, (2000), Family therapy & alternative medicine: Acupuncture as a case in point. *Contemporary Family Therapy*, 22:1, 3-18.

— — —, (2000), Spirituality as a component of health care, Best Practices. *Working Together: the Family Collaborative Health Care Association* Newsletter, 5:2, 4.

— — —, (1994), Reflections on "being there" and "doing" in family therapy: a story of chronic illness. *Family Systems Medicine*, 10:1, 99-110.

— — —, (1992), Creating a network of volunteer resources in a psychoeducational family asthma program. *Family Systems Medicine* 10:99-110.

CPSIA information can be obtained
at www.ICGtesting.com
Printed in the USA
FFOW05n1751011014

9 781936 778485